The Art of Healthy Living

'Denise Kelly's *The Art of Healthy Living* is ... f fresh air in the health and wellness industry. The boo ... rves as an easily digest ... or creating and s staining a life of balance, joy, and ... ng. Ideas and concept. ... down so beau ... fully through the use of storytelling ... our th ... don't even ... much I am abs bing until the end of each chapter ... ind of ... ok I will revis ... again for knov dge, inspiration, and motivation fr ... expert ... er field '

Ross King, Television and Radio Presenter, Actor, Producer and Writer

'Having met Denise a few years ago we immediately had a connection – and our connection was illness leading us to find health through what we put in and on our bodies. My awakening came in 1991 when I changed my relationship with food and how and what I ate. Denise has had a similar experience – her story is inspiring and thought provoking. This book explains it all and shows how the achieve optimum health and happiness. For those starting out on this journey I recommend this fabulous book! '

Jo Wood, Former Model, Television Personality and Entrepreneur

'I thought I had a relatively healthy diet and a good outlook on life, but Denise Kelly's insight and knowledge of the world of health, wellbeing and nutrition have opened my eyes. Just making a few small changes can make a really big difference to anyone. I'm personally excited to start making them! Thank you, Denise, you are an inspiration.'

Laura Hamilton, TV Presenter, Mum and Entrepreneur

'This practical guide to healthy living is a must for anyone who wants to improve their mental state, physical energy or emotional balance. Denise presents her ideas in a practical, informed and inspirational way that makes healthy living easy and fun.'

Steve Neale, Speaker, Trainer, Psychologist and Coach,
Co-author of *Emotional Intelligence Coaching*

'I hate patronising self-help, "I'm-so-great" type of books – this is NOT one of those. Denise writes with humour, kindness and realism. Her approach is passionate, warm and genuine, but most importantly EASY to understand and very enjoyable. There will be something in this book that will resonate loud and clear to every single one of you. I personally have a good knowledge of the importance of nutrition, exercise, and being outdoors, and so wasn't expecting to gain too much – how wrong could I be? No one knows it all, and if your life is even just a little bit shit, you should definitely read this. If your life is completely shit, then look no further, Denise will aid your recovery (whatever your problem or problems are) and potentially turn your life completely around. It's a book that will warm your kitchen; nurture your bedside table and cuddle your soul. I have read it all, but I will forever keep to hand – for reference, guidance, recipes, medical grievances, encouragement and support. Every household should have a copy: in fact, it should be the law. Thank you, Denise, you are an angel.'

Frankie Park, TV Presenter, Model and a very firm Believer in all round wellness

'*The Art of Healthy Living* is perfect for anyone looking to achieve the right balance in life and wanting to 'thrive!' What I loved is that this is not simply a book about nutrition and fitness, but it's also about the mind, our emotions and the thoughts we allow to enter our mind daily. In other words, it's about it all .... BODY, MIND AND SPIRIT. It's personal, it's passionate, it's "spot on" ... with a detailed road map for anyone to follow. I live and work in NYC... It's a phenomenal city... But it's often stressful, chaotic and challenging... One needs balance. Denise Kelly clearly and simply outlines how to achieve and maintain that Balance. An essential read for a lifetime!!!'

Michael Christie, Entrepreneur

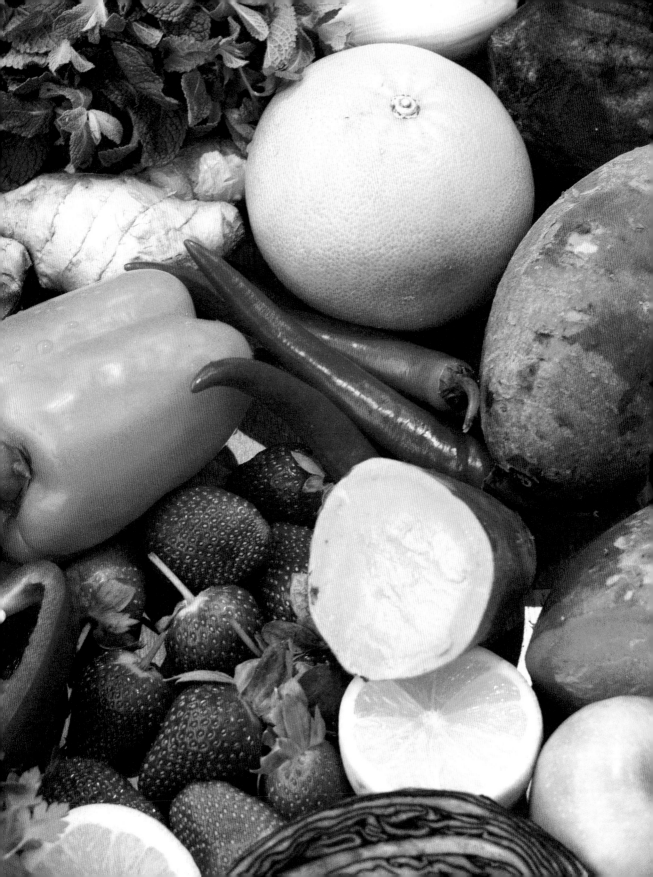

THE ART OF
HEALTHY LIVING

How good nutrition and improved well-being
leads to increased productivity, vitality and happiness

Denise Kelly

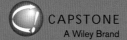

CAPSTONE
A Wiley Brand

This edition first published 2020
© 2020 Denise Kelly

Registered office
John Wiley & Sons Ltd, The Atrium, Southern Gate, Chichester, West Sussex, PO19 8SQ, United Kingdom
For details of our global editorial offices, for customer services and for information about how to apply for
permission to reuse the copyright material in this book please see our website at www.wiley.com.

Library of Congress Cataloging-in-Publication Data
Names: Kelly, Denise Naturopathic nutritional therapist, author.
Title: The art of healthy living : how good nutrition and improved well-being leads to increased productivity,
vitality and happiness / Denise Kelly.
Description: Hoboken : Wiley, 2019. | Includes index.
Identifiers: LCCN 2019024529 (print) | LCCN 2019024530 (ebook) | ISBN 9780857088116 (paperback) |
ISBN 9780857088185 (adobe pdf) | ISBN 9780857088178 (epub)
Subjects: LCSH: Self-care, Health. | Nutrition. | Health—Psychological aspects.
Classification: LCC RA776.95 .K45 2019 (print) | LCC RA776.95 (ebook) | DDC 613.2—dc23
LC record available at https://lccn.loc.gov/2019024529
LC ebook record available at https://lccn.loc.gov/2019024530

A catalogue record for this book is available from the British Library.
ISBN 978-0-857-08811-6 (pbk) ISBN 978-0-857-08818-5 (ePDF) ISBN 978-0-857-08817-8 (epub)

10 9 8 7 6 5 4 3 2 1

Cover design: Kathy Davis/Wiley   Cover images: Courtesy of Bailey Sadler

Set in 10/14pt FrutigerLTStd by Aptara Inc., New Delhi, India
Printed in Great Britain by Bell & Bain Ltd, Glasgow

The opinions in this book are Denise Kelly's own, and do not reflect the opinions of John Wiley & Sons
Ltd. This book should not be used to diagnose or treat any medical condition, and should not be used as a
substitute for the advice of a qualified Medical Practitioner.

CONTENTS

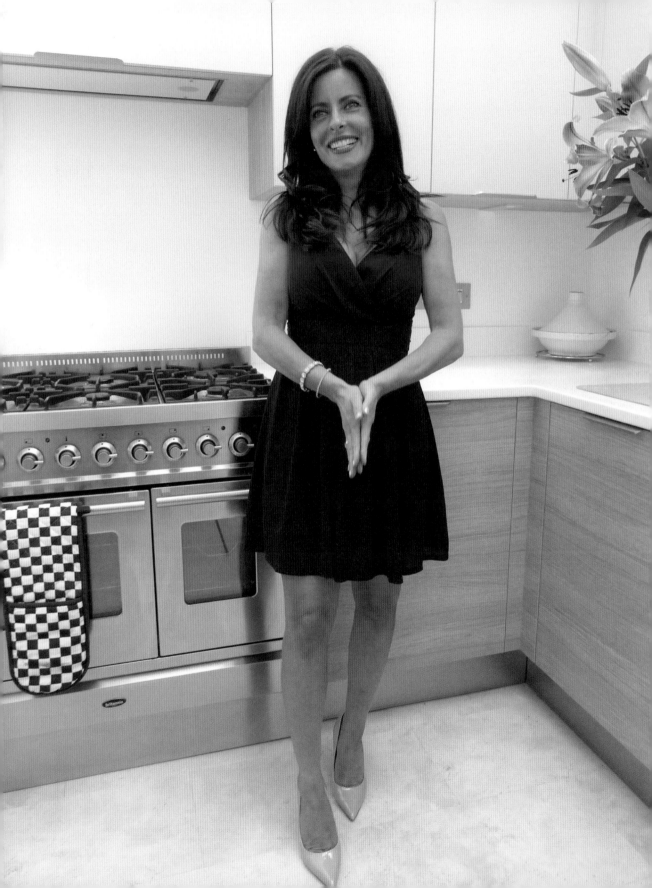

CHAPTER 1

KEEPING THE BALANCE

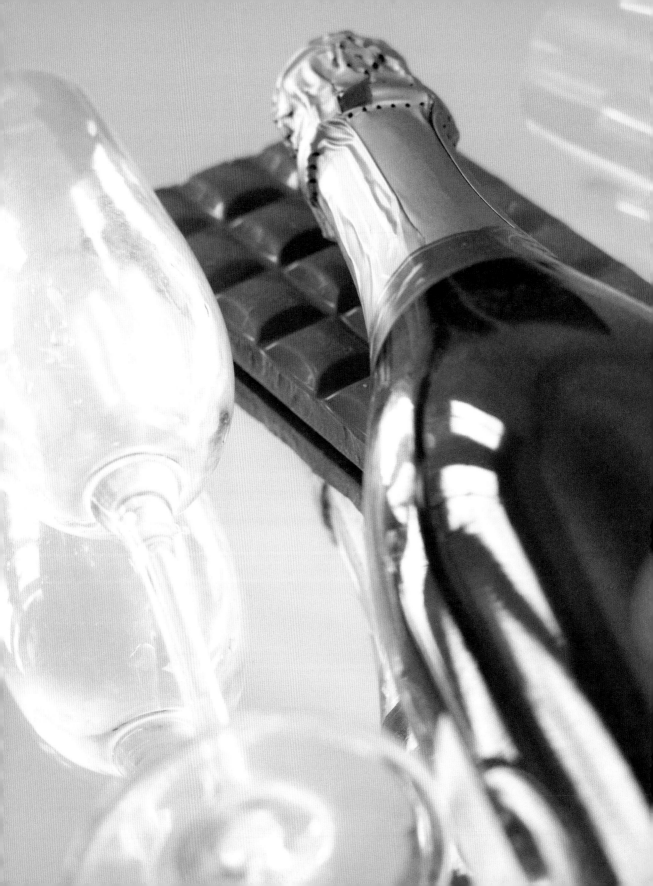

I like prosecco and I like chocolate. Not the opening lines you would expect to read when you find yourself embracing your new 'nutrition to create success' book! By the way, I do also love juicing and eating fresh whole foods.

To me, this is the secret to good health and success … yes it's all about the BALANCE!

Getting a happy balance of life is vital, and this of course means many things, as I will explain. Firstly, looking after yourself nutritionally, buying the best quality foods you can find, not eating processed junk, and not downing a bottle of vodka every day of your life is pretty important. Trust me, in my experience as a nutritionist, I have just about seen it all in my clinics over the last 15 years (drug addictions; miracle cancer stories; sleep disorders; digestive complaints; heart attacks; liver, kidney, and bladder disease; allergies; strokes; asthma; mental, physical, and emotional disorders; daily depleting migraines; anxiety; hormonal disorders; diabetes; osteoporosis; arthritis; infections; deteriorations; fatigue; injuries … and the list goes on and on!).

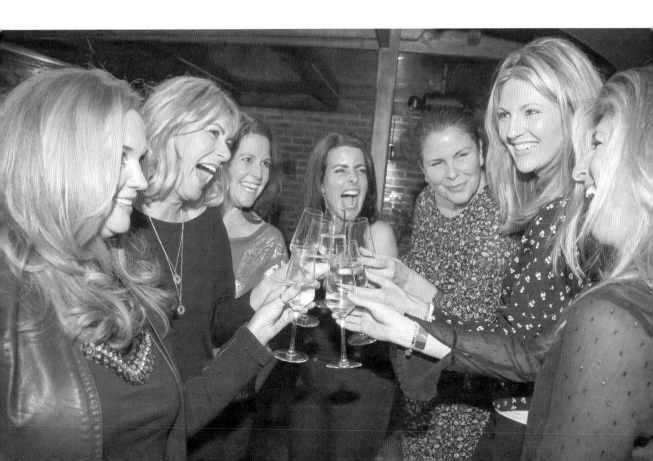

I have found that being happy with your life, including all aspects – work, relationships, and success – is just as important as what you are eating and how much exercise you are getting. However, it is a vicious cycle: it goes without saying that the healthier you are, the more strength you have, leading to more energy. Higher energy creates much better behaving hormones, happier and more uplifted feelings, and a more positive general attitude. It also contributes to greater brain power with more clarity, calmness, and focus. When you are focused and in control of your emotions and your life, you make better decisions, which will help you move forward in the way that your heart desires and create passion, success, and achievement in all areas.

Life is short, right? There is no replay, so live it to the fullest.

After all you only get one shot (I know everyone has different beliefs, but that is irrelevant right now, because you really do get one shot at being you, right now, in this lifetime) so why waste time feeling pants? If you are not fuelled correctly, you will feel tired all the time, lethargic, low in energy, maybe even a little depressed, foggy in your thoughts, and unmotivated. Maybe you catch colds really easily, or you have to take a course of antibiotics each winter season because your body just can't cope and you spend wasted hours in bed feeling poorly? Or maybe you are suffering from an illness that you know you could help if you had a better diet? Migraines for example can be completely debilitating for some people and cause endless sick days. From my experience, and the way I have worked with many clients over the years, you need to clean up the condition of your blood, clear the toxins out and strengthen your liver function, and the migraine attacks will disappear. None of this is rocket science. Sometimes the simplest of things can completely turn your health around and give you back that incredible zest for life. It's just down to knowledge and informed choices.

How would you feel if I asked you to create an existence for yourself that you truly love? Doesn't that make the most sense? I meet so many people every day that dislike their jobs, or have fallen out of love, but they are hanging in there because they are scared to be alone, or struggling with debt, abuse, or not achieving their goals and feeling despondent and disappointed with life.

Well, I am here to tell you, with conviction in my heart, that you can, and you will, turn your life around if you really have the desire. Knowledge is power and once you know, it is up to you what you do with that information. You can lead a horse to water, but you can't make him drink!

Also, when you are newly equipped with information, it's really easy to want to tell everyone that you meet and lecture them with your new-found knowledge that's going to change the world. I was like that when I first qualified as a nutritionist, and when I look back now I feel utterly mortified! I thought I knew it all. But of course, I didn't. It has taken years to understand what works and what doesn't and that everyone is different. We all have our own journeys to go on in this world of discovery. Some people

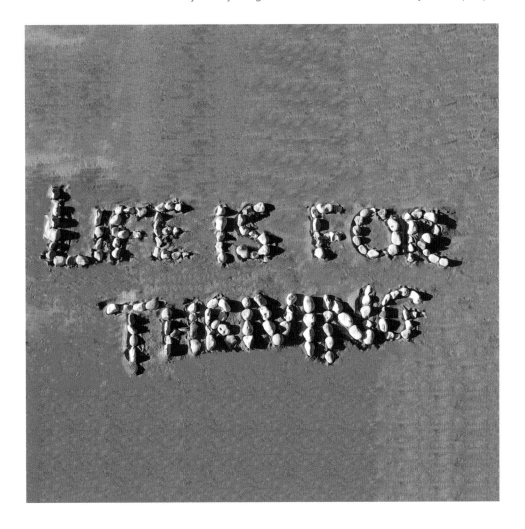

are just not ready to hear information that could propel them into success, or a happy relationship, or becoming a leader, or the best parent in the world!

Changing the way your body feels and making yourself stronger and more desirable is a dangerous place to be … because it moves out of the comfort zone of 'stuck' and into the unknown zone of 'amazingness' and 'anything is possible'. The sky is your limit, and this can be a very daunting place, believe it or not! The best way to share your knowledge is to lead by example. If you look amazing, ooze confidence out of every beautiful pore in your skin, and are glowing with enthusiasm and vitality, I can guarantee you that people will want a piece of you. Then, and only then, should you share your knowledge. Why? Because they want to be just like you!

So, you can party, you can eat out, you can drink a little if that's what you like to do, but inform yourself how to put your body right the next day, and the day after that, until it's so ingrained in your life that living this way becomes normal. You can get such a high from eating 'clean' that you will want less of the 'bad stuff' and be high on the more beneficial energizing foods that I am going to tell you about throughout this book.

My motto in life is: 'Life is for thriving, not just surviving, and why would you want it any other way?'

CHAPTER 2

BELIEVE AND ACHIEVE

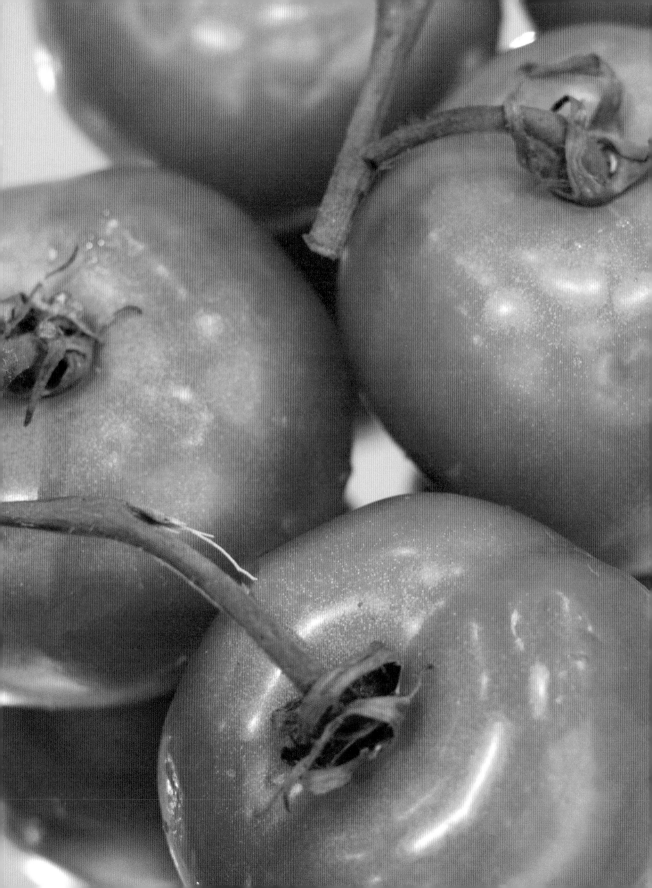

My passion for health began in the year 2000 when my beautiful baby girl was born. Up until that point I had been relatively healthy all my life. No major illnesses and naturally in good shape. I was one of those that pretended to go to the gym, but really spent the entire time chatting to everyone and not doing much else! Shortly after my daughter was born, I started getting stomach cramps, to the point where, every time I ate, I felt nauseous and unwell. While all my friends that had babies were desperate to lose weight, I was shedding weight at an alarming rate. I had always been a curvy girl, as a teenager and in my twenties – an average UK size 10. I had boobs and a butt and was proud of them!

As the pain continued, and the weight fell off I reached out for medical help. Having grown up in a healthy family, with an average life expectancy (from the grandparents) of around 90 we didn't go to the doctors much. My parents believed in homeopathy and we saw therapists for reflexology, acupuncture, and reiki if we felt unwell. So it felt kind of alien to me to have such problems that wouldn't go away. That year I saw three gastroenterologists, had tubes up, in, and down to look at every angle of my intestines and they found nothing.

Don't get me wrong, I think doctors are amazing. I have doctors as relatives, and know they perform miracles every day, working with the information they have, but in my case they couldn't find out what was wrong. Having a newborn child would have been exhausting at the best of times, but I was up half the night doubled over in pain, unable to digest anything, and feeling tired and afraid. As regards my daughter, it is as if she knew, from the day it all started, how to behave in a way that was overwhelmingly supportive to me. From just six weeks old, she started sleeping through the night and has never been a moment's trouble ever since.

So now, I had gone from a healthy size 10 to a skinny size 4–6. I had lost my curves and I didn't feel like me at all. The doctor actually told me to go home and eat a 'good pie', but how could I when I literally felt like everything hurt? Telling me there was nothing more they could do gave me no option but to seek 'alternative' help. It's a pattern that I am all too familiar with now, as most of my clients don't see me as their first port of call. They see me because they are running out of options and are desperate to feel well. I like to spread the word that prevention is better than cure, but I guess not everyone sees it that way.

I trawled through the internet and tried to find a practitioner that I thought might be able to help me. I started reading about Ayurvedic medicine and eventually booked myself an appointment with the most incredible practitioner. It's to her that I owe my passion for my career. When I saw her, I was 29 years old, skinny and frail and desperate for help. She told me my condition was simple to fix and that once I had learnt from her how to use food as my medicine, I need never be in pain again. She was right … and it changed my life.

I remember looking at food in a completely different way. I started looking at every single thing that went in my mouth as something that would help heal me. Sure enough, over the next few months my appetite returned, the pain disappeared, and I felt happy and energetic again. In my eyes it was incredible and I wanted to learn more.

After my amazing son was born a year later, I decided I wanted to study naturopathic nutrition. I thought it would be a fantastic thing to know and could help my family immensely. If I could bring my children up knowing how food could make them feel, and teaching them to eat well, it would be a life skill they would have forever. I didn't really see past that, and certainly had no idea that it was going to turn into the unbelievable career that I have today. However, before it was really going to fully blossom, life was going to throw another few little curve balls my way … DEATH and DIVORCE! Oh how it doesn't rain but it pours.

Separating from my husband, with two young children, was without doubt one of the hardest and most painful things I have ever had to endure. I remember sitting on my kitchen floor just after he drove away for the last time and honestly thinking my life was over. The first few months were a bit of a blur and I could feel myself slipping slowly down a slope of self-destruction. I was not in check with my emotions in any way, as I was so struck by grief that all my thoughts were being utterly hijacked and disoriented. Being the party girl that I was (pre children) I thought it seemed like a very good idea to go back down that road. WRONG! What it did for me was make me feel lower than I had ever felt. My mind was going crazy, my body was getting depleted and I looked tired, haggard, and hopeless.

Even though I did know how to take care of myself at this particular time, I was choosing to ignore that knowledge. While I was in that state of mind things were only going to get worse. I had children, other family members, friends, a dog, and a home to take care of and it wasn't pretty. My little secret mission was to apply my make-up every day and face the world with a smile on my face. If I could make each day without a total meltdown it would be a miracle. I would do the school run, walk the dog, get the grocery shopping, meet friends for coffee, go to work and make everyone else feel fabulous and healthy, all with a perfect smile and newly mascaraed lashes (always waterproof for the silent tears in the car journey between each task). I became so super-good at pretending and faking it I should have received an Oscar for the ongoing per-formances I put on over the years that followed. During the divorce I lost friends, family, and at times my sanity. Money was tight, the mortgage was high, and I was drowning in a pool of despair. I thought I could bag a new husband by fluttering my eyelashes and being entertaining and funny, but inside my heart felt dead. Why oh why was everyone else on the entire planet happy except me?

When you look back at yourself in your worst moments its insanely ridiculous that we do this to ourselves. Drink to excess, party, and have fun! Fake fun! So many people choose these destructive routes. It's called avoidance and denial and it needs serious attention.

Sometime later the unimaginable happened. Fairly soon after my own grieving period, one of my best friends – someone who had talked me through the worst few months of my separation and helped me with endless advice on how to earn more money and get stronger once my husband's income diminished – chose to take this destructive route. We had been friends since the age of two, and although very different characters, we had a massive amount of love for each other. She was my daughter's godmother and a beautiful larger-than-life character that everyone adored. For her, the drinking, the parties, the lack of sleep, and a pretty out-of-control existence quickly led to serious and fluctuating levels of anxiety and clinical depression. Her situation became much more frightening and after just over a year of this constant self-destruction she actually took her own life. It was devastating to everyone that knew her, and something we could never have imagined would happen. Do I believe she would ever have done this in her right frame of mind? No. Never. She was the most successful person I know, she had love in her heart, and a soul so clever she could connect with anyone. She was successful beyond most people's wildest dreams (awards from Richard Branson and the Queen for her contribution to London business) because people loved her. She believed in giving everyone a chance, and if they proved themselves, they were 'in'. She achieved more in her 45 years than some achieve in a lifetime.

The point is, the body is incredibly robust, and is actually your best friend.

It will literally do anything to try and keep you well and hundreds and thousands of communications are going on between your beautiful cells right now to help you read this book, digest your food, and aid your memory so you might just remember some of the things you read! But, if you abuse your body over and over again, with drink, drugs, processed foods, and sleepless nights eventually something will go wrong. I believe that all disease is a result of our lifestyle choices, and I don't just mean the food that we eat. If we are continuously unhappy, have issues from our past that we are avoiding, and know they are affecting everything about our future we need to seek help, seek therapy. If you know you are unfit and it's affecting your daily energy and your enjoyment of life, get a personal trainer. If you don't have enough money, go running or go for a walk. It costs nothing. If you have an illness that is causing you pain, discomfort, challenges and hindrances, get a nutritionist. There is always a solution, no matter what your problem is.

For myself, I had some knowledge. I knew that my destructive ways were undermining my body, and that I had to face up to the reality of what was going on in my world. I loved my children more than life itself and it was they who got me out of bed every day and gave me the strength to go on. But my heart was broken and so was I. At this point I had choices to make. Enough was enough. I felt weak, vulnerable, and an utter failure. The only way from there had to be up.

I knew that, in order to take some of the pressure off myself, I had to start earning more serious money. I had debts to pay off and a life to provide for my children. So I started writing a health column for a local newspaper to create a wider audience and gain clients. This worked brilliantly and I have not had to spend a single penny on advertising since. It has a weekly readership of 70,000 people and very quickly I started getting regular emails and began to build a real rapport with my readers.

Because of this I began seeing more clients on a regular basis in three different clinics in the UK. This also gave me a platform to promote health and well-being talks and presentations. At one of these local events a wealthy businessman happened to be passing through town. He was sitting in a coffee shop and opened the paper at the page that my column was on. There was my announcement about the health talk I was giving that evening. Unbeknown to me, he was an entrepreneur who travelled the world teaching managing directors and CEOs about emotional intelligence and being a leader that works from the heart and not from the head. He had for some time been looking for a nutritionist that would be able to travel with him as part of his masters training programme.

My talk that night was in a nearby hotel, and I had sold around 60 tickets. There were about five spare tickets, but I always had a few extras turn up on the night, so it all seemed good. It was a relatively small venue and I was comfortable with my subject and felt quite relaxed about the evening. What I always hoped for from these events was that I would inspire people to live healthier and happier lives and inform them of the best ways to look after themselves nutritionally. Off the back of this I would then gain new clients who perhaps knew they needed more specific help with their health. Finally, I was about to discover that my luck was beginning to change, in a big way … Halfway through the first session I could see out of the corner of my eye a sharply dressed guy walking into the room. Not only was he coming in late, but he sat directly in front of me in the front row. I didn't recognize him, but I certainly noticed him, almost to the point of being distracted from my flow.

At the end of the first half I suggested to the audience that they could buy juices and smoothies (a separate business I had created, alongside my clinics, with one of my best

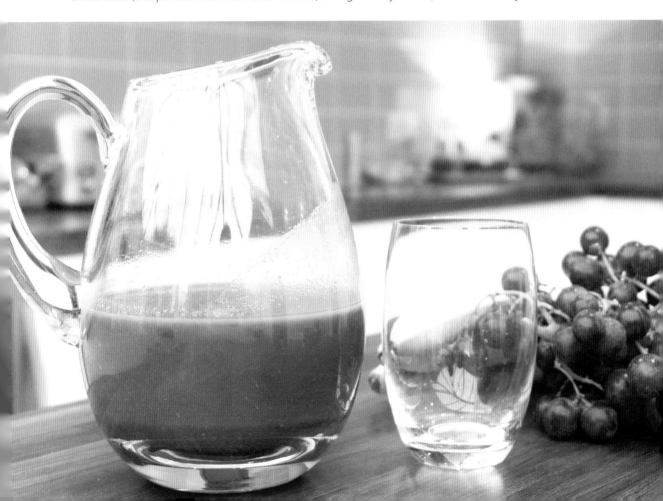

friends) and told them to feel free to come and talk to me if they had any questions. This was always a popular moment as the people attending usually had some sort of illness or ailment that they wanted advice about, which I was always happy to give. But this well-dressed, polished looking guy that had come in late leaped out of his seat and headed straight for me before anyone else had a chance. Handing me his business card he said: 'My name is Steve, and I run a corporate training company teaching large groups of business executives how to lead through emotional intelligence. I have been looking for a nutritionist to teach alongside me to inspire these people to eat properly and gain energy through their diets. I have been looking for two years, and now I have found you. I want you to come to Lithuania with me next week to start training them. I will pay well, book your flights and cover all your costs while you are there. Call me tomorrow with your answer.'

A week later I was on a plane to Vilnius, in Lithuania. Once I arrived, I had to catch an internal plane about an hour inland. It was the middle of winter; the snow was falling heavily, and the plane was tiny … and it had propellers! I boarded the 1950s-style plane thinking 'I have literally lost my mind. I am about to die in a country I know nothing about, am meeting a man I don't know in the middle of nowhere and I have never trained anyone in the corporate field in my life. I have no idea what I am doing, and what if they all think I am rubbish and don't like what I have to say and … blah, blah blah! I want to be back at home in my warm house, with my children, snuggled up on the sofa!' Someone get me oooouuutttt ooooffff hhhheeeerrreee!!!

Turns out it was the best decision I ever made. Those few training days had forced me to step out of my comfort zone and changed everything about my business and how I valued myself. No longer was I the local nutritionist, I was an international jet-setter giving lectures all over the world about a subject that I was so passionate about – I could talk about it for hours and hours. For days on end! Well, I wasn't quite there yet, but what this man saw in me was something I hadn't even seen in myself. He believed I was capable of delivering what he needed in less than 10 minutes of knowing me, and now, so did I.

I think, looking back, that when you have hit rock bottom, there is an inner strength that you can find, that comes from nowhere. It's like a survival mechanism that suddenly rears its head and says 'you must start to get your shit together!'

I stopped drinking and started putting into practice all the things I had ever been taught. I ate only foods that I knew were going to uplift me, heal me, and keep my energy and

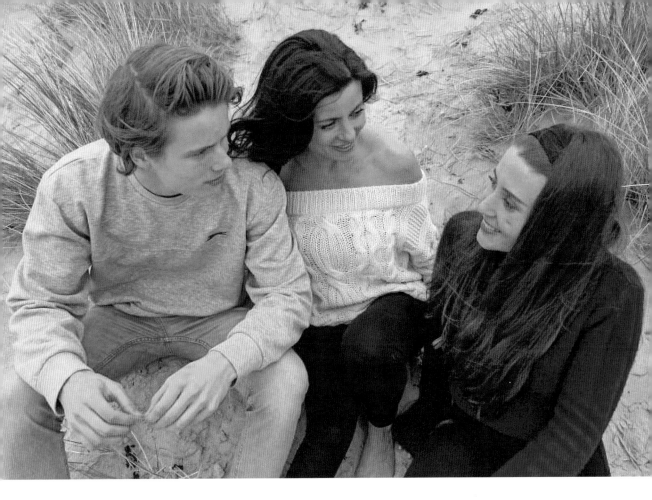

mood high. I started to practise yoga and meditation on a regular basis, and ran further and faster every day. I joined more fitness classes, drank green juice … and slowly but surely the dark clouds began to lift.

Digging deep into your soul to regain your strength is not an easy task, but it's a mighty rewarding one. What doesn't kill you does make you stronger. With the utter love of my children, my parents, my sister, nieces, and best friends, I started to feel lucky again. Before, all I looked at was the negative. I had no husband, friends had deserted me, and I was financially broken. If I didn't turn this around things were going to get bad. Once I started to feed my body the correct fuel, I began to see the value in small things and feel grateful for everyone that had stood by me in my darkest days. I realized that I may have fewer friends now, but at least I know who my true friends really are. Surely it is about quality not quantity. The friends that would call me every day and constantly make me laugh though the tears. The friends that would force me to run every morning even when I was exhausted. My children for loving me beyond anything I could ever imagine and giving me a reason to get out of bed every day. My parents who loaned

CHAPTER 3

GET YOUR DUCKS IN A ROW

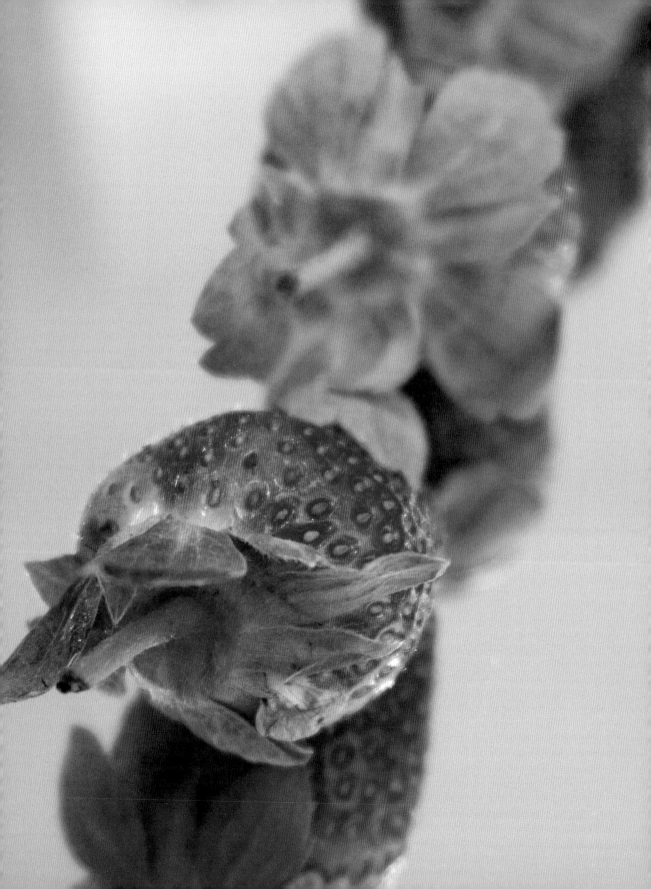

Whatever is going on in your life you need to find the strength to keep your health robust. Whether you are feeling fabulous already and just want to learn more in order to maintain that, or you have hit a life crisis such as a bereavement, divorce, loss of finances, loss of your job, heartbreak, addiction, etc. Or maybe you have great ambition and wish to climb the ladder of success, and know you are going to need a shedload of brain power and energy in order to achieve such things. If your health is resilient and strong, it's surprising what you can cope with.

If you have any stress at all in your life – and most of us do in one way or another – you need to raise your 'health-enhancing game' and put all your efforts into keeping your energy and vibrancy high. When your body is stressed it needs all the nutrient-rich foods it can get. Imagine an intravenous drip of goodness filling your body with the best vitamins and minerals nature has provided. That is what I teach my clients to do daily, and the results are phenomenal. I don't mean endless supplements and pill-popping, so you are rattling as you walk down the street. I mean good old-fashioned whole foods, superfoods, juices, and smoothies. If you power your body with these life-enhancing foods, it does not mean that you will simply forget about your problems, or that your heartache will go away. It just means you will have the power to deal with them without collapsing in a burnt-out heap in a year from now.

When you go through an emotional time in your life, your body goes into fight or flight mode. This is OK temporarily, as our bodies are designed to warn us if there is danger lurking. Your breathing will become faster, your body will release stress hormones to cause your blood vessels to constrict and divert more oxygen to your muscles, so that you have more strength to take action. But this raises your blood pressure and elevates the cortisol levels in your body, which, over a prolonged period of time, can interfere with your learning, memory, immune function, bone density, and cholesterol levels. Your nervous system releases a truckload of adrenaline, which sends your body into a hyper overload. With the crazy-ass pace that most of us live at, this intense level of stress will eventually start to affect your sleep, leaving you feeling depressed and despondent. Your digestion will suffer in all areas: bowel movements, acid reflux, etc. (In Chinese medicine, your digestion is the root of your health and if that goes out of kilter you are in trouble).

This has the potential to send your hormones into overdrive affecting fertility, sex drive, and moods and can cause increased feelings of unhappiness. Your skin becomes dry and ages more quickly, your hair and nails can thin and lose that beautiful shine. Not to mention the extreme seriousness of how it can rapidly weaken your heart. Apparently, when your heart is broken, perhaps in the case of a bereavement or lost romance, it almost doubles your risk of a heart attack or stroke. Emotional stress can kill. So while taking care of yourself might be far down the list as you deal with your stressful situation, looking after your health should be your number one priority!

If you look at someone and they are gorgeously glowing, they have a huge smile on their face, and positive words seem to just flow out of their mouth, how attractive is that? Someone who exudes health and vigour is going to be noticeable. If you wish to change something about your health, your life, and your mindset, you have to put in the groundwork. If you are an entrepreneur, or you want to climb the ladder of success in life/business (and that will mean something completely different to everyone) it is vital that you get your ducks in a row and work out what you need and when. Like anything in life, it doesn't just land in your lap. Some of us are born with a naturally stronger constitution than others and come from a stock of 'good genes' but even you – and you know who you are, because you brag about it over a pint at the pub – are at risk if you don't look after yourself properly.

My background training was in naturopathic nutritional healing. This means that my learning includes many different health systems utilizing a variety of different treatments in order to get well. I chose that path because I do not believe that one system alone is a cure for all. I like to understand many different elements of health that have spanned thousands of years before us, because although we have the most incredible medical advances that save lives every single day, I have my personal views on why so many people are so sick nowadays and, scarily, my own age bracket (forties) and younger are by far the worst that I see. The forty-somethings and below have the most toxic bodies I see in my clinics and they are the most stressed and those with the least amount of genuine energy.

What I mean by genuine energy is not the kind that's fuelled by coffee, tea, or energy drinks. That is fake energy and the biggest mistake you can make when you are tired and exhausted is to reach for stimulants. When I visit companies, if there is a glass office and I am having a meeting in there, the number of people I observe refilling their coffees during a two-hour period is alarming! I don't think coffee itself is actually bad. Just ensure, as with all food and drink that you purchase, that it's great quality, but moderation is key. In my opinion just one or two cups a day is ample if you love it, and there is research to show that it can have health benefits such as positively helping in the prevention of Parkinson's disease, type 2 diabetes, and liver disease.

However, if you are a stressed-out bunny, feeling like you will hit the deck if you don't have your caffeine fix, mark my words: you do not need that extra cup. Why? The overuse of stimulants when you are already stressed to the max will weaken your immune system, create cravings for high salt and sugar foods, aid weight gain, and completely crush your ability to handle any stress whatsoever. Even remarkably simple tasks such as deciding what you are going to have for dinner that evening could potentially create feelings of anger, uneasiness, and anxiety and be completely overwhelming. Basically, if you feel like this you are in 'anxiety overload' and your emotions will be like a ship in a storm. In that case it would be wise to make different decisions about what you are putting into that preciously fabulous body of yours.

I remember once in the 1990s being on a ship crossing the Atlantic from Portugal to San Juan, Puerto Rico, in 30-foot waves. Almost the entire ship, including me, had to have injections in their buttocks to stop the continuous throwing up. The lifts were full of vomit, as were the corridors, the cabins, and the beauty salon. It was quite a scene! And that will be the analogy of your life if you choose to stay in adrenal overload. I don't mean you are literally going to be vomiting uncontrollably in random corridors. But your life will be chaotic and out of control. If you think this is you, do not fear, all is not lost because with the correct balance of foods and nourishing drinks you will bring yourself back into line, and it may not take as long as you think. This is the beauty of what nature gave us. It's all here, ready for us to take full advantage of to help regain our balance. It's remarkably clever!

When it comes to helping make a person well, I like to apply all sorts of considerations when dealing with disease. For example, Chinese medicine considers the laws of nature, the environment around us, and the natural physical response of the nervous system to help create harmony. They see the body as a whole: not only defined by the organs and systems it carries, but also as the home of the mind and spirit. Have you ever noticed when you travel on holiday you feel a certain way? Different in mood? Maybe more relaxed? More peaceful or happier? When you are in a different environment your body uses different organs to properly respond and provide for your needs.

Also, when the seasons change, our bodies need completely different types of nourishment. It's so important to remember that the body is an extremely powerful instrument. Its intelligence works far beyond the capacity of the human brain, and in therapies such as acupuncture, herbal medicine, homeopathy, and reflexology, the basic principle is that the body is smart enough to heal, once it is given a reminder of its own fabulous functioning. In acupuncture, for example, when the needle is inserted the reality is that it's invading your body. Your entire nervous system is woken up and goes into attack mode. The good news is that during this process your body gets a jump-start and the areas of weakness in your body get a little shake-up – a wake-up call to start moving. So areas of blockage, or stagnation, or inflammation begin to heal. You see it's not actually the needles that are healing you at all, it's your very own nervous system as its starts to create a natural regulating and healing process from your blood getting a boost and starting to flow properly.

The body is like a gentle river and needs to be constantly flowing freely in order to be healthy and for you to feel your best.

If there is a blockage anywhere it will initially try to come in. At first you may not notice, as it's just lurking in the background, but pay more attention to it and you will begin to be alerted to the problem. Your body is trying to protect you and the problems come in the form of pain, swelling, acid reflux, nausea, seeing blood or an unusual discharge, or other forms of discomfort. This is your body letting you know that danger is lurking, things are changing, and the problem needs to be solved. The quicker you solve it, the better. If you know you have something that feels uncomfortable and it's not usual for you to feel like this that's your body telling you loud and clear something is wrong and you should take notice. In our Western world we ignore so much. We immediately reach for the painkillers, the digestive pills, the blood pressure tablets. All we want is a quick fix. Unfortunately for all you quick-fixers out there, there is NO magic pill to keep you healthy. Meditation, yoga, regular exercise, practising gratitude, being thankful, eating clean, avoiding processed junk, being kind, seeking herbs and therapies to aid your suffering mind are all part of the picture for maintaining your lifetime of wellness and health.

The one thing that drives me crazy is when people think this type of life is boring! I am not saying for one moment you have to give up all the things you love. NEVER! I am the most un-nutritionist you will ever meet. Come party with me and I will show you! Drink your alcohol or eat your treats if that's your thing … but if you know how to rein it in and keep it clean for the majority of each day you are going to feel totally in control of yourself, your life, your emotions, your sanity, your body shape, your body tone, your ageing genes, your greying hair, your spreading midriff, your saggy boobs, your drooping bottom, your eye bags, your breath, your teeth, your bones, and your muscles.

To be fair, the people that usually say to me 'I would rather die having a good time, than have a life of eating lettuce leaves' are usually the ones that have the most health problems

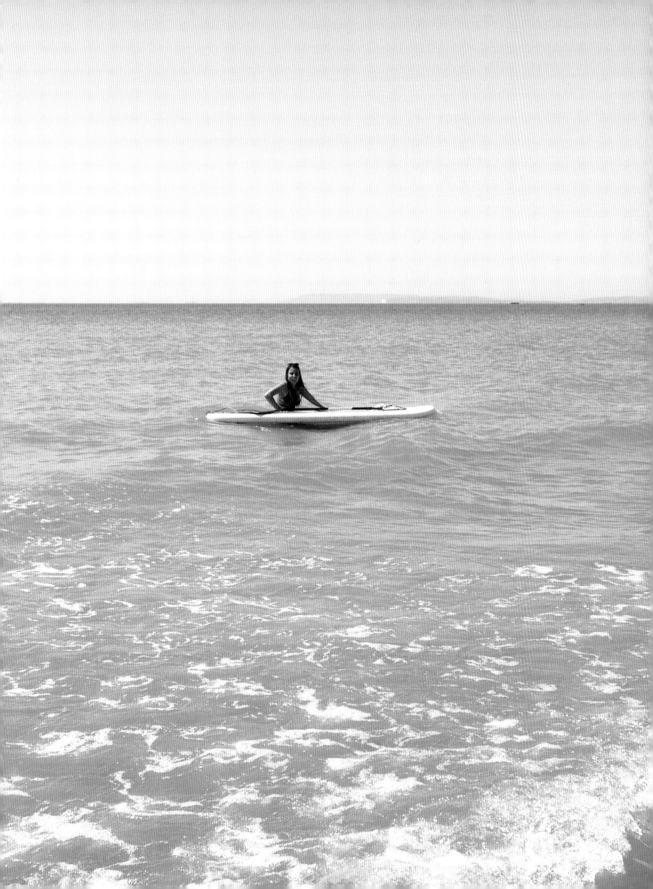

and need to make the most changes. After all, we are often resistant to the things we need the most. Trust me, when you have been eating clean for a while and removed all your toxic substances, you will understand what I mean. You suddenly have so much energy you literally don't know what to do with it. What's that film where the guy takes a mysterious pill that enables him to access 100% of his brain's abilities? Bradley Cooper stars as a struggling writer who, because of his new-found intelligence, becomes a financial wizard. This puts him in a new world of success and danger, but also offers considerably more excitement to his life. That's it … Limitless.

If you get the chance to watch it, I would highly recommend it. The comparison I am trying to make here, is that a life with true health and energy makes your life 'limitless'. When you have enough physical and mental energy you can do whatever you want. All your ambitions, hopes, and dreams become far more reachable. Your every waking thought is more positive, and life becomes a magical journey of untold discovery and bravery. The better you feel, the more you do. Your confidence grows and so does your zest for life.

The Secret

If you are familiar with *The Secret* you will understand that positivity creates and breeds yet more positivity. This best-selling book written by Rhonda Byrne was released in 2006. It's based on belief in the law of attraction, which claims that the thoughts we have every day can completely change a person's life. It has sold over 30 million copies worldwide and been translated into 50 different languages. Its central idea is that everyone has the ability to create their own reality and that 'thoughts become things'. The seven laws of attraction are widely used and I talk to my clients about them all the time as I feel they can be massively influential in setting your mind on the right path of positivity. The first is the law of manifestation. This means that anything we focus on constantly will manifest in our lives. So, you negative ninnies out there that think you are down on your luck and nothing good ever happens to you … well of course it doesn't, because you always think it's going to be bad. This is the number one rule in our house: don't focus on your problems, just focus on your dreams.

Fight the Negativity

When I was going through my divorce, I spent three years focusing on all the things I didn't have. *Three precious frikkin years* manifesting a shitball of badness. And that's all I got. Stress, worry, financial loss, crappy dates, awful fallouts, and tears like Tiny Tears on acid! Crying, moaning, hysteria, drama on a loop that went on and on and on. It wasn't until I realized one day that I was surrounding myself, and just about everyone else that came into contact with me, with endless negativity that something had to change, or my life was going to be this hellhole existence forever. I was going to die in a pool of black sludge called self-pity!

I rarely have any regrets in my life. I feel like everything I have ever done, good, bad, funny, naughty, ecstatic, sad, horrid, lovely, has all been one big learning curve leading to now. But I really do regret wasting three solid years of my life on something that could have been resolved in a calmer and more pleasant way, and possibly much more quickly. I am, by my own admission, a very 'passionate being'. When I feel that I, or my family, have been betrayed or wronged, or that someone has behaved unjustly, I'm very unlikely to let that pass. As I mature, the 'passion' or the 'fire' is lessening, or perhaps I am simply more reasonable. These days I am far more grounded and try with true empathy to see situations from all angles. Now I listen to friends who sadly find themselves in the situation that I was in and try to advise them how little the small things matter and not to enter into the fight. But it's their journey to learn from, so they may or may not be ready to listen. It's the same when it comes to health. We cannot force, persuade, or dictate to anyone about getting their health back on track. Even those who can easily avoid suffering may not be ready to hear what you have to say.

The second law of attraction is the law of magnetism. Meaning that we can only attract the same kind of energy that we put out about ourselves. Our personal energy moves outwards from us and connects with others of like resonance, which, according to *The Secret*, determines both who and what we attract to ourselves in life. The people and situations that are drawn into our lives match our signals. Is it chemistry? Or more of a resonance, a matching signal due to personal vibrations? It's a harsh reality, but if you don't like the society, partners, friends, or success that you have attracted so far, or you have found real difficulty in finding your 'place' in the life that you desire, you will seriously need to consider what you are putting on your calling card to the world. I guess the good news is that since this frequency is something you produce yourself, it's definitely something that you can change. Your personal resonance is created through your vibrations and your feelings and your emotional energy. It's also crucial to change the vibrations of the very thoughts that go through your head every day if you know they are negative. Just because other people can't hear what you are thinking, doesn't mean you are not emitting them. Your physical energy and the vibrations of your body are crucial because us humans can pick up instinctively on how we think someone is feeling. Negative thinking is usually based on three fears:

1. **Fear of the future:** Even though it hasn't happened yet, so logically why should we be afraid?
2. **Fear of rejection:** That inner voice that says we are not good enough, unlovable, not clever enough, etc.
3. **Fear of failure:** Why bother trying, right? We will just fail anyway.

Even as you say all this to yourself, you can feel your body sinking, can't you? All fear is toxic to the energy of achievement, so it's clear that when we think this way, we are creating our very own self-fulfilling prophecy of doom. These negative thoughts destroy optimism and are our greatest challenge to overcome in reaching genuine happiness.

The other laws of attraction include unwavering desire, which is your constant and unwavering passion for a certain outcome. In other words, your total belief that this is what will happen. And the law of delicate balance, the law of harmony, the law of right action … in other words, making things happen in order to achieve your goals. So, for example, not taking action in the right direction for your nutritional goals would be … you have a sore throat and a cold and you feel terrible. To boost your immune system you could juice ginger, lime, oranges, cucumber, and garlic three times a day until your body has soaked that up and feels better again. But instead you choose to eat fast food, drink two bottles of wine, and feel shocking the next day, making your body even more tired and toxic, giving you five days feeling miserable in bed! You see how your choices and actions can seriously affect your outcome.

The final law of the universe is far greater and more powerful than just you, but equally as important for achieving happiness. Understanding that we are all 'One' with each other and the entire universe is the foundation law. I am a believer in karma and living a good life that you are open about and proud of. Speaking your truth sets you free and trusting your own desires makes you who you are. The long and short of this is that every area of your life, including your health, your finances, and your relationships, is influenced by 'like' attracts 'like'. Everything you may want or not want to experience is pure energy vibrating at different frequencies. The basic premise of the law of attraction is that energy attracts like energy. Whatever you are vibrating out there to the world, you get right back. Things that you long for or desire will not come to you until you are sending out the right vibrations for that to happen. So, don't blame, simply change.

Change your thoughts, your visions, your mindset, your negative chatter, your beliefs, your needs … and see what happens.

The more we, as human beings, understand about the way we work, what we need, and how things unbalance us the better equipped we are at really making a difference to our lives, our health, and our overall well-being. Not only does this understanding have an impact on our own minds and bodies, it also helps us to understand and have more empathy for others.

Ayurvedic Medicine

Ayurvedic medicine (developed over 3000 years ago in India) is another favourite of mine that really helps a person to understand what they are and why. It shows clearly that if you slip out of balance your life can really spiral out of control. The theory behind Ayurvedic medicine is that good health exists when there is a balance between three fundamental bodily humours or doshas (the three energies that define a person's make-up). Each human body is different and the way Ayurvedic medicine explains this is that each person has a unique blend of physical, emotional, and mental characteristics. Because of our body type, each one of us has slightly predisposed weaknesses or strengths, and if we know and understand this and can feel ourselves getting out of balance, it is easier to correct. The three body types are vata, pitta and kapha. I am going to outline the main traits of each one, just so you have a basic understanding of what you need.

Vata

The vata-type person is generally speedy. They are vibrant, quick-thinking, creative, fast-talking, dynamic, and slightly airy people, but they can also be very sensitive as well as spiritual and are often running late. (Stop shouting at the book, anyone that knows me! Yes, yes I have a lot of vata qualities!) Vata-type people can be fidgety, forget to eat, and generally routine can feel awful, boring, and overwhelming to them. They are usually thin in appearance, with delicate bone structure, low body fat, and they often find it hard to gain weight. On the flip side when this person is out of balance, they can be indecisive, stressed and prone to what I call 'burn out', exhaustion, and fatigue. They can have thinning hair, lots of gas and bloating, and can be very unfocused and spacy. They can also have dry nails and skin and are the types that need to wrap up as can feel the cold easily. They suffer from sleeplessness, excessive worry, and vitamin and mineral deficiencies.

I think it's useful to understand this concept because it gives you more empathy as to why some people act the way they do. Without doubt, it has helped me to understand my clients better and may help you to understand yourself and what your needs are in order to maintain balance. What a vata person needs is constant nourishment of the nervous system. They need to take extra special care of their digestive system, as well as looking after bone strength and protection. Vata types need to stay away from low fat foods and must be careful if vegetarian to stay grounded and nourished. They need warming, heavier foods to stay calm, good quality oils and good fats, and strengthening foods like mashed sweet potatoes, root vegetables, black and wild rice, lots of fish and eggs and heavier grains such as buckwheat. Vatas can get great results from exercise such as weight-lifting, Pilates, and yoga.

Pitta

The pitta body types on the other hand, tend to be very fiery, determined, confident, and can at times seem aggressive. When out of balance pittas can be dictatorial and easily angered. They have a medium body frame, are well-proportioned and can be muscular; they tend to have good genes. They are compelled to accomplish things and can therefore be extremely focused and organized. You will not find a pitta type missing a meal, purely because they can actually be really cranky if food is skipped, and most pitta types will know this about themselves and try to avoid this situation. They can be workaholics, and don't always do well in hotter humid climates. Emotionally they can create problems that don't really exist, and sometimes even when they are feeling too balanced! They have the capacity to work until they drop, which is not advisable, as they then spend time and effort picking up the pieces. Pitta types are ridiculously organized, energized, enthusiastic, and sharper mentally than a vata. However, out of balance they are easily agitated, irritable, and desperately over-competitive. Physically they can suffer with diarrhoea, skin rashes, burning eyes, increased appetite, perspiration, and have a greater need to nourish their livers, gall bladder, spleen, small intestines, and blood than the other body types.

Foods that will be beneficial to a pitta type are sweet tasting spices, cardamom, fennel, and proteins such as chicken and fish. They need lots of dark leafy greens, and peppermint tea. Fresh limes are particularly good for them, and they need to be careful and make sure to reduce excessive spices that are too heating. Heavier red meats are not great for them at all as they dampen their energy. They need calming and relaxing physical exercise such as yoga and Pilates, and from an emotional perspective, they need gentle relationships. This is very interesting if you are married to a pitta person. They won't respond well to ranting!

Kapha

The kapha types are generally larger bodies, not necessarily overweight, but they can have a tendency to gain weight easily. They are usually strong and robust characters and when in shape can be powerful and athletic. They are usually very grounded people, who are solid and stable and clear about the ways of the world. They are strong sexually and have a slower metabolism. They can miss a meal, unlike the pitta types. They are much more resistant to exercise and are generally slower moving, often trying to lighten up, both physically and emotionally. They are reliable types, dependable and calm and can be peacemakers, even-tempered, loving, and affectionate. However, when they are not in balance, they can hold onto emotions, bear grudges, and feel depressed and despondent. They can sleep too much, lack enthusiasm, feel dull, sluggish, overweight, and congested and can be the least enthusiastic of the types if they allow themselves to live incorrectly.

The organs which most need to be nourished in this body type are the lungs, stomach, body fat, and lymphatic system. Heavy and high fat foods, dairy, gluten, red meats, and starchy vegetables are all a no-no for this type of body. They are best suited to beans, quinoa, spinach, salads, cayenne pepper, ginger, and heating spices. They need positive affirmations daily and good amounts of cardiovascular exercise.

It's interesting when you read this information for the first time, because in your head you are now categorizing everyone you know. I would just add that you are not necessarily going to be only one body type – it is very common for you to have a combination of two. For example, I am a classic combination of vata and pitta and have those exact traits if I go out of balance. What helps, though, is that when you understand a little bit more about the differences between us as human beings, it can make you look at people in a different light, with far more love and understanding for what they are and what they need.

Many of my clients who are fifty-plus years old seem to have better health than the generation below. I am generalizing here, because of course there are very healthy people in the younger age category too, but from what I have witnessed the oldies are generally cleaner! Internally! My generation and below have been exposed to far more junk and processed foods than ever before. Ready meals in some families can be the norm, as can fizzy drinks and diet foods. The quality of meat is not so good, our fruits and vegetables are laden with pesticides and other chemicals, and sugars are everywhere, in everything.

Alcohol consumption is at an all-time high among teenagers and some of my clients in the professional and corporate world drink excessively due to the nature and socializing aspect of their jobs. Many of my clients (and friends) are, perhaps without realizing it, functioning alcoholics. Drinking too much alcohol on a daily basis has all sorts of effects on your health. It can increase your chances of developing cancer, cause stomach distress, thin your bones, change your coordination, alter your behaviour, distort your mental clarity, shrink your brain, damage your heart, cause pancreatitis and infertility issues, not to mention creating malnutrition, increasing diabetic complications, and severely battering your poor, very important, liver. If your liver is damaged it can prevent the removal of harmful substances from your body, leading to a backup of excessive toxins, undoubtedly leaving you feeling PANTS!

Health should be your most prized possession and you should treasure it. Look after it every day. Do not take for granted that it will always be there for you, running in pristine order, because I have seen all too many times how devastating it can be when something goes seriously wrong.

I have given many talks in corporate settings about health and well-being. I can always tell from the outset who has been forced by their boss to come to my 'well-being day' and who is happy to be sitting in front of me. I can see the almost childlike look on faces when I start to talk, as they are looking at their watches and thinking 'I have got so much to do and don't want to be sat here listening about how to be healthy!' These people normally have the body language giveaway … they are slumped in their seats, heads down, perhaps biting their nails or fiddling with their hair, looking out of the window. Hand on heart, I actually love seeing these people turn up under the boss's orders in an attempt to get the whole company interested in how to live healthier lives. To me it's a challenge. As I talk, slowly but surely I can see something that I have said finally resonate in their brains. Perhaps I have made a connection with a disease that their mother suffered from, or talked about a client who has turned their life around from severe challenges to vibrant health, or spoken about mental health issues and they feel exactly the same, but just haven't told any of their work colleagues yet. Their body language begins to change. The posture straightens out, their necks elongate like a peacock looking for a mate, they start to make eye contact with me, maybe even raise a little smile, their heads tilt to one side as they wonder how they are going to make a difference in their own lives, and maybe even those of their family. It is the people that looked the least interested at the beginning that are the ones queueing to see me at the end with a list of questions so long I could be there for years giving answers.

When I first started out, I was always very nervous to be in the 'corporate world' giving health presentations. Everyone seemed to be so powerful and super-successful. But strip that back, and client after client revealed to me that it doesn't matter what you do, how high up in your organization you are, how many promotions you have had or how many bonuses you've received. Take your clothes off and stand there naked, remove the title and the flash car and mansion house, and we are all the same. Everyone has their own insecurities (and if you say you don't you are telling porky pies). Everyone has their life scars, their emotional baggage, their fears, phobias, and health issues. Everyone has wobbly bits, or too-skinny bits, or more cellulite that they would like. We are fundamentally all the same. It is best for us all to create good health in order to enjoy life to the fullest, and enjoy doing all the things we want to do. So let's keep it simple and keep it real. We need good food in order to feel amazing, and of course a whole heap of other stuff thrown into the mix.

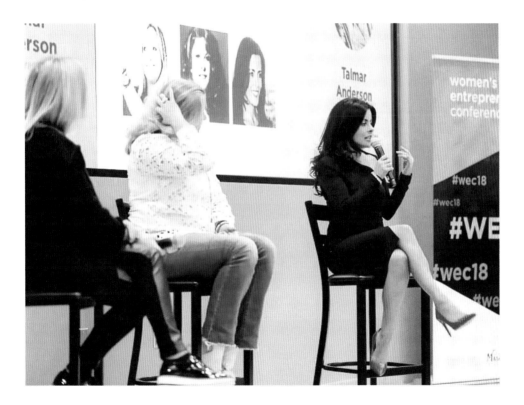

Maybe you are stuck in a toxic relationship or surround yourself with negative people who suck the life out of you, or you're with someone who thinks its clever to make you feel utterly worthless, in order to elevate themselves and their own ego. What do you do? You, my friends, need to work on yourself. You need to build your strength up in order to get out of the kitchen (so to speak)! Well, hopefully you are going to be in the kitchen doing a lot more preparations, as you need to get super-strong in order to create and raise your vibration. You attract exactly what you are putting out there. It's as simple as that. In order to know how much you are worth, or to change yourself to be a better version of you and get rid of any life-sucking vampires or change your own negative thought patterns and behaviours, you need to get in control of yourself, your life, and your health ... pronto.

Life is very unpredictable, people come into your life, situations change, challenges occur ... so be ready and fully equipped. Whether you have a family or not, the person you need to take the most care of and rely on is yourself. You are far better for all your loved ones if you are in a good physical, mental, and emotional state of being, and the chances are you might be a much nicer person to be around too. Put in the work and the rewards will be magnificent. The stronger and more robust you can make your body, the better you will be in every way. The more vibrant you become, the more you can cope with, so when you are faced with a stressful situation, or a complicated dilemma, or a heart-wrenching blow to your trust in humanity, you are ready to take it on ... head on!

The glory comes from daring to begin!

CHAPTER 4

CHANGE THE SIMPLE THINGS

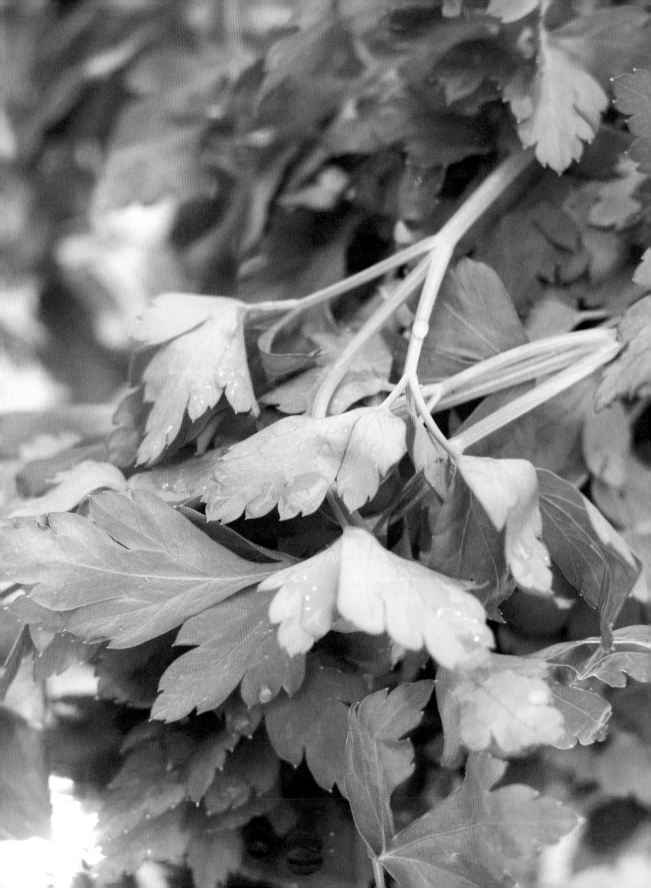

Sometimes it's the very basic things we have far more control over changing that can offer us the biggest impact on how we feel. It is these small changes that make a profound and lasting difference.

Good health generates many things, and what I want to make perfectly clear is that I do not profess to know everything there is to know about nutrition. It is a minefield out there and information changes every day, as I am sure you are aware if you've ever tried to search something health related on Google. Quite frankly it could scare you to death just reading that stuff! One minute there are trends and everyone's on the bandwagon for a certain type of diet that is a cure for all, and then a year later it's going to kill you! I have so many confused clients who say they don't know what to eat and what not to eat.

What I can share is over 15 years' clinical experience with clients from all over the world, with just about every ailment known to man, and the basic ingredients to gain better health the way I know it. One of the most important lessons I know to be true and one that I share regularly is *do not wait for your alarm call*! Do not wait for something to go wrong in your body before you start really taking care of your beautiful brilliant self. Prevention is far better than cure and the slope to wellness is a small incline rather than Mount Everest. On the other hand, if you are suffering and you have the drive and/or need to get well, there is so much hope. When you have hope you have everything, and one of the reasons I love talking to large audiences is because so many people do not realize how possible – and sometimes dare I even say 'easy' – it is to get themselves back on track.

The question I ask everyone is this: 'How would you like to look and feel every day?' Energetic, happy, glowing, calm, healthy, focused, vibrant, and in control are amongst the many words that get thrown back at me. We all want to look and feel our best all the time, so why not create a life where you can be just as you wish. You will have down days, hard days, feel not so well days, but if you knew the basic ingredients to gain back your health, correct your hormones, make your digestive system function normally again, rid yourself of migraines, diabetes, and muscle aches and pains, then surely you would do whatever it takes?

Often new clients they can be quite resistant to change. The number of people that are completely terrified to sacrifice what they love to get well is surprising. In my experience it is not so much down to willpower, but addiction, be it sugar, alcohol, bad fats, etc. It's not necessarily the person's fault, well not directly anyway. You see they are often so deficient in minerals and vitamins that the only way they think they can feel any better is to eat what they love. So when they eat five chocolate bars a day, initially they get a high and feel better, and then they crash. I will explain more about the importance of maintaining balanced blood sugar levels later. The way I would work with a client that has these types of deficiencies and addictions is to remove very little from their diet in the beginning but add the good stuff instead. When I do eventually ask them to cut down or remove completely a food that they thought they adored, it is then less of a struggle to take away that particular food because they are nutrient rich, and their bodies are feeling naturally more satisfied.

I am guessing you realize that the body system is pretty complex? If you sit down and think about every process that's going on in your body right this very second it will probably freak you out. The human body is literally a miracle and I find it incredibly fascinating. Almost 99% of the mass of the human body is made up of six elements: oxygen, carbon, hydrogen, nitrogen, calcium, and phosphorus. Only about 0.85% is composed of another five elements: potassium, sulphur, sodium, chlorine, and magnesium.

> ### *The human body is made up of over a 100 trillion cells and each and every one of those beauties wants to do its best to look after you.*

Cells are the basic building blocks of all living things. They provide structure for the body, take in nutrients in the form of food, convert those nutrients into energy, and each one carries out specialist functions. They also protect the body from toxic invaders and try to keep us safe from harm. Your cells are amazing! And you need to look after them.

Being well equipped with good fuel is essential before you can start to feel improvements in your willpower and va-va-voom. There are some extremely easy things you can do almost instantly to change your mood. If you implemented these few things into your daily regime the difference it could make is enormous. Also, if you are going to do something and you fully understand why you are doing it then that particular thing is going to be so much easier and less challenging. Remember knowledge is power!

Hydrate Yourself with Water

Yes, I know you know this. It's obvious and everyone talks about it, but do you actually know why we need to stay hydrated? Even a small decline in your body's hydration can make things very difficult for you. Straight away your focus starts to weaken, you can feel dizzy and confused, your heart can beat in weird rhythms, and you can begin to feel tired. Your concentration levels decline, and you can feel low in mood and energy. Some people experience headaches, and a dry mouth, but whatever your symptoms, you need to know that being dehydrated is bad for anyone and everyone. If you suffer from allergies such as asthma or hay fever you need to take even more care of hydration. Dehydration causes the body to produce more histamine and asthmatics have excessive levels of histamine in their lung tissue which can cause bronchoconstriction and increased mucus build-up in the lungs, making the airways more restricted.

If you suffer from allergies, being dehydrated will also make symptoms such as coughing, sneezing, and runny eyes and nose worse.

Water is God's wine! Whatever your beliefs it's as natural as it comes and water is really the only drink we should be having throughout the day if we want gorgeous skin, incredible brain power, better circulation, fabulous digestion, greater absorption, and more excretion. Yes, if you are constipated it's quite possible this is why. You don't have to reach for over-the-counter medication. You simply drink more water and eat more fruits and vegetables. I've seen so many people in my clinics over the years that are chronically constipated when all they need is more fluids (fruits and vegetables are sometimes as much as 96% water). Not having regular bowel habits can cause all sorts of havoc in your gorgeous systems. Your skin can get breakouts as the toxins back up in your body, you can get puffiness around your eyes and even skin rashes. You become bloated and uncomfortable and lose your healthy appetite. It can also give you bad breath and a bad taste in your mouth resulting from overgrowth of toxic gut bacteria which work their way back up right into your mouth. Yuk! Stress is also a major factor for constipation but staying well hydrated can really help.

Try not to reach for drinks that will dehydrate you further, such as fizzy soda, beer, wine and spirits, hot chocolate, coffee, sweet tea, and energy drinks. If you don't like plain water, then why not add something healthy to make it taste more refreshing, such as lemons, limes, mint, ginger, or cucumber? Lemon in water provides extra health benefits such as adding vitamin C which is a primary antioxidant that helps protect cells from damaging free radicals. It helps reduce your risk of cardiovascular disease and stroke and lowers blood pressure. It aids your digestion, flushes out your kidneys, and helps prevent kidney stones. It can also help keep your liver clean, which is essential for the optimal functioning of your body. It can improve muscle and joint pain and encourage natural bowel movements, which will make you automatically feel lighter and more energized.

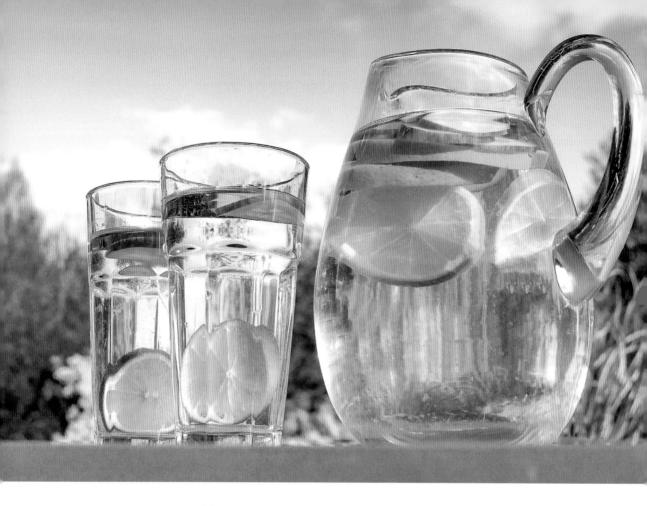

NOTE: Never add extra sugar to your water with citrus fruits, as this is a potential dental disaster! If you are worried about the enamel on your teeth try drinking through a straw.

Limes have virtually the same benefits as lemons; it's just a case of personal preference. Both are acidic outside of the body but help to balance our bodies' natural pH when consumed internally. How much you have depends on personal taste, but the juice of even one a day will have benefits such as reducing the risk of some types of cancers. Recent studies have shown links between citrus fruit consumption and diminished risk of oesophageal cancer, although more research is required but it's definitely food for thought. Limes are also high in antioxidants and can help with the appearance of your skin. The limonin found in limes can help prevent the accumulation of streptococcal bacteria, so including limes in your daily water may help stop these harmful organisms from developing and prevent bacterial illnesses.

Cucumber in water is not just for your spa day anymore. It has real health benefits and if you are not slicing these green gems daily and adding them to your H2O then it's time to start. It helps prevent cell damage as it's rich in vitamin C, beta-carotene, manganese, vitamin K, magnesium and vitamin B1. It's great for your muscles, helps transport calcium to your bones, amazing for your skin as it contains silica, and helps lower blood pressure due to the potassium content. It boosts weight loss as it can curb your appetite due to the high number of vitamins and minerals it contains; therefore it can leave you feeling more satisfied than just water on its own.

Not only does mint add a great flavour to water, but it has many health benefits which extend much further than just digestive help, although the benefits for this are immense. Mint is thought to increase bile secretion and encourage bile flow, which not only speeds up and eases digestion, but also supports healthy cholesterol levels. It can also help relieve pain and discomfort from gas and bloating; in addition, it contains an anti-inflammatory agent called rosmarinic acid which helps with pain and inflammation, both topically and internally, and can also improve allergy symptoms.

Fresh ginger root contains active enzymes, so helps massively in relieving nausea and settling most stomach complaints including vomiting. It helps to regulate high sugar levels, soothes the stomach, and improves absorption of the nutrients and minerals.

You can even have a 'flat tummy water' recipe!

For 6 cups of filtered water –

1 teaspoon grated ginger

1 cucumber sliced

1 lemon sliced

1/3 cup mint leaves

Let the mixture infuse overnight and drink the next day!

Water is amazing! Your 100 trillion cells need it.

There are no hard and fast rules on how much you need as there are differences of opinion. I would say it depends on your size and weight, your activity level, and where you live – if the climate is hot or cold, etc. The general rule of thumb is that 8 x 8 ounce glasses (which equals about 2 litres per day, or half a gallon) can be consumed. This is called the 8 x 8 rule and is very easy to remember, although if you know you are the type of person that drinks nothing, then build up slowly increasing your amount week by week. It is a fantastic habit to get into though. Try it today. If you get that afternoon slump, instead of reaching for the biscuits, reach for the water and drink a full glass. The difference it will make to how you feel and how your brain functions is extraordinary. You become alert, awake, and brain-energized once more. So, add those lovely natural flavours to your water, and do anything you can to get it down the hatch!

NOTE: Try to always drink water from a glass bottle and not plastic. Plastic is dangerous and harmful to your health because BPA (a component found in plastics) is a hormone disrupter that has been linked to hormone imbalances, toxicity, inflammation, and even cancer. There are dozens of other chemicals that are potentially dangerous too, affecting the endocrine system and fertility and increasing toxicity within your body. You can buy glass bottles from all major supermarkets now and it's the safest way. Normally, when your bottle undergoes any type of temperature change, whether it's in the car and the car gets hot, or it's put in a fridge to get really cold, that's when the chemicals can leach out. Everything is about choice, and not only is glass a better choice for your health, it's also a good environmental decision.

 WARNING

I have a friend who refuses to drink plain water but adds squash to everything she drinks. This is a *big* NO NO!! Squash drinks are complex and sugar-free squash even more so. The ingredients are usually water, sweetener, aspartame, or sodium saccharin, juice in a low quantity, large quantities of flavouring, preservatives, and colour such as anthocyanin.

NO NO NO! This is *not water*!

You must understand that this will not have the same cleansing effect as plain water with the natural flavours in. You are adding substances into your body and you know nothing about their effect on your health. And it's unnecessary. I have said it before, and I will say it again: your tastebuds will change, and you will start to enjoy the less man-made sweet treats, and it won't take long for that to happen. Just give it a chance! Water is by far the best and most anti-inflammatory drink in the world!

Eat Some Fats!

Think Mediterranean! Olive oil drenched over tomatoes and garlic! Mmmm! No wonder people who live there, live so long! Let's get one thing clear … eating fat does not make you fat. At least not the good fats. Let's get a good perspective on what is a good fat and what isn't. For years I have had people telling me they cannot eat nuts or avocados because they are on a diet, but they can eat some no-nutrient slimming bar with a heap of rubbish in. The message is so wrong! You know as well as I do that if you sat there night after night gorging yourself on bacon, sausages, burgers, pies, cheese, cream, butter, pastries, cakes, and biscuits you would feel sluggish and gain weight, not to mention raise your chances of a heart attack. The reason that that men over 45 and women over 55 are far more likely to have a heart attack than their younger counterparts is because, over time, plaque build-up thickens and stiffens artery walls, which can inhibit blood flow through your arteries to your organs and tissues. The most common cause of heart disease is atherosclerosis, and *it is correctable*.

I was at a seminar recently listening to a cardiologist talk about the problems we face as a society in relation to heart disease, and how preventable so many heart conditions are. People could avoid life-threatening surgery if they only addressed a few things such as unhealthy diet, being overweight, smoking, or lack of exercise. Four things! That's it! This is not rocket science and it's not hard to know what contains *bad* fats. Have you ever cooked bacon, and left some on the kitchen side for a few hours where the dripping fat hardens to room temperature? It's a solid white mass of yuck. And that is what is settling in your beautiful artery walls, when they should be free flowing … just like the river I told you about. Without flow, we do not *go*!! Did you know that the World Health Organization has classified processed meats – including bacon, salami, ham, and frankfurters – as a group 1 carcinogen. In other words, there is strong evidence that processed meats cause cancer. At last, after years of research they have finally come to a conclusion that people may listen to. The government is now under pressure to add labels to these types of meat in the same way they had to put warnings on packets of cigarettes about the dangers of smoking.

There are so many things I could say that are important if you are going to start making changes to your diet in order to improve your health. Taking away the bad fats and including good fats in your regime is one of the very best things you can do. Fat is a crucial part of your diet and this should be one of your health goals every day. If you avoid fat altogether you will cause damage. Each and every beautiful cell in your body is crying out for you to ingest fat! But so often, day after day, it's deprived and depleted. I see it with my clients all the time. The good fats are known as essential fatty acids and are beneficial and vital for our well-being.

Have you ever suffered from any of the following?

Constipation, dry skin, weight gain, low energy levels, brittle hair and hair loss, poor nail growth, deterioration of liver and kidneys, depression, inability to sleep, low immune system, digestive issues, inflammation and bloating, allergies, and low libido? The chances are you are very deficient in good fats.

The human body cannot make omega 3 on its own so you've got to lend it a helping hand. Without it, you will not function properly. The 100 trillion cells I keep banging on about rely on omega 3 in order to do their job properly in forming a healthy membrane that surrounds each cell. Your cells have to be permeable in order to let the good stuff in and the bad stuff out, and also to perform millions of other functions in your heart, blood vessels, lungs, immune system, hormones, endocrine system, brain, retina, and sperm cells. I treat more people now than ever before for infertility issues, and this is one of the first things I will talk to them about.

Remember, if you have healthy cells, you have a healthy body. Simple!

It is suggested that we need between 250 and 500 milligrams daily of omega 3 to function optimally. It's found naturally in fish such as salmon, tuna, herring, sardines, and mackerel, and other seafoods, but we have a massive problem with polluted water, which makes fish perhaps not the best choice anymore. So you need to find healthier alternatives. Fats are found in abundance in nuts and seeds, such as flaxseeds, chia seeds, and walnuts. Also plant oils such as flaxseed oil, soybean oil, and canola oil. Algae supplements also have good supplies. It's essential to get a good supply of these fats because so much can be affected in your body if you don't. If you include omega 3 in your diet it's going to be a huge help in protecting you from cardiovascular disease, cancer prevention, Alzheimer's disease, age-related macular degeneration, dry eye disease, and rheumatoid arthritis, plus many other ailments.

Omega 6 fatty acids are also essential, so you need to obtain these from your diet too. These fats are primarily used for energy. Although omega 6 fats are essential we have to be careful not to consume too much of them. I know, it's so confusing! The reason

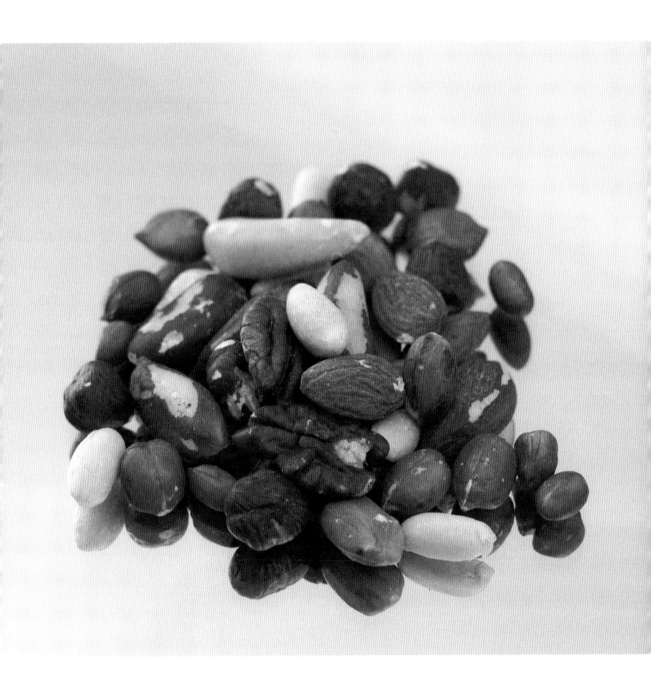

for this is that these fats have been known to increase inflammation if you consume too much in comparison to omega 3. The recommended omega 6 to omega 3 ratio is 4:1. Before we relied so heavily on processed foods, we consumed them both in equal measures. When we eat from nature, as we were intended to, we got what we needed from the plants, algae, nuts, and seeds and our bodies were clever enough to distribute it as they saw fit. I think our deficiencies and incorrect ratios have a great deal to do with the rise in asthma, coronary heart disease, cancer, autoimmunity, and neurological disease, as they are all believed to stem from inappropriate inflammation in the body.

I would suggest that the best plan is to follow an anti-inflammatory diet, based on plants and wholefoods that are more alkalizing to our systems. Our bodies are super smart but need help if we are to survive in this Western culture. We walk into a supermarket and everything is presented so nicely, and the packaging tells us that its 'healthy' and 'good for us', and the dieters amongst us see 'low calorie' this, and 'sugar-free' that. It's like showing a magpie shiny objects continuously.

We are drawn to things that look great, when actually what we really need to be doing is taking everything back to basics.

If we want to eat fish, go catch it; if we want to eat cake, go bake it; if we want to eat fruit, grow it; if we want to eat vegetables, plant them. This is something I am very passionate about. So many people that I have seen over the years have turned their health around simply by eating what our grandparents and their parents before them were eating. Cut out the fast food, the take-aways, the white bread, the crisps and chocolate, and voila … your body could just start functioning properly again!

Omega 6 is just as important for our body functioning as omega 3 – protecting the heart, for example – we simply don't need quite so much of it. The healthiest food choices to get omega 6 are flaxseed oil, hempseed oil, grapeseed oil, and pumpkin and sunflower seeds. Also pistachios, pine nuts, borage oil, evening primrose oil, and acai berries.

So, to set this straight, the body needs omega 3 and omega 6 fatty acids, but cannot make them, which is why we need to eat foods which contain them and why they are called 'essential'. Omega 9, on the other hand, is described as 'non-essential', because our bodies can synthesize it from other things that we eat. Omega 9 may benefit your health by helping to lower the bad cholesterol and raise the good and may also play a role in helping to control blood sugar. The foods these fats can be found in are olives, extra virgin olive oil, sesame oil, avocados, and nuts such as almonds, pecans, cashews, pistachios, hazelnuts, and macadamia nuts. All these help to keep the body in good balance.

The benefits of including omegas 3, 6, and 9 are endless. They can increase our energy and stamina, help decrease cravings, and burn calories. They prevent heart disease and decrease inflammatory disease such as arthritis. They can massively help with inflammatory bowel disease, hormonal function and PMS. Your brain is over 60%, so what do you think is going to happen if you increase your consumption of the right fats? It's going to improve your nervous system, help alleviate any feelings of depression and memory lapses, and make you feel alert and positively clever! They also assist in transporting minerals that keep bones and teeth strong, helping to prevent osteoporosis, and have antifungal properties, staving off infections. Not only that, they regulate gene expression which in turn inhibits tumour growth. And as far as beauty goes, if you want to stay looking young, get on the omega-popping bandwagon, because without it you may gain a few more wrinkles! It has been proven to give you clearer, younger looking skin, strong nails and shiny hair. And it's a lot cheaper than Botox!

Quick Fact About Fats

Fats such as butter, margarine, and lard become toxic once heated or exposed to light or air. It is suggested that coconut oil is perhaps the safest fat to cook with, but it's debatable whether there are any other oils that are meant to be solid. It's also worrying that many oils are sold in plastic containers, which have been proven to leak toxins from the plastics into the oils. The containers do not protect the oils from the light or the heat either, making them extremely unhealthy. Research has been done on this subject that suggests this could be contributing to degenerative disease. At the same time, other research has been done linking high-quality, cold pressed omega oil blends with the prevention and recovery from degenerative disease.

These are some other recommended oils:

Udos Choice: this is a carefully chosen blend of omegas 3, 6, and 9 in the correct ratios. It contains active lignans, antioxidants, and anti-inflammatory elements and benefits every cell in the body.

Coconut oil: this has undergone quite a bit of scrutiny recently. Personally, I love it, but it's like everything, use in moderation. If you are an athlete, you can consume more; if you have a very sedentary life, you need very little per day. I think it has many health benefits, such as helping to lose fat, better brain function, killing bacteria and viruses, and it can be used as a beauty product to moisturize the skin. It helps the absorption of other nutrients, although I would not suggest you eat it to excess, as it does contain a type of fat that can increase cholesterol levels, but at the same time it does have fabulous anti-oxidant properties. Coconut oil helps boost your metabolism, giving you more energy throughout the day and eating it straight from the jar can actually help anti-inflammatory issues such as arthritis. It is classed as a superfood because of its many benefits. You can also use it to cleanse the mouth and treat gum disease by a method called 'pulling'. This involves swishing a tablespoon of oil in your mouth on an empty stomach for up to 20 minutes. This action supposedly draws toxins out to improve oral health, but it is said to be beneficial for general health too.

Blue/green algae: when you consume algae foods such as chlorella, spirulina, and E3Live you are essentially eating what fish eat and therefore getting all the minerals, enzymes, and vitamins you need as well as an abundance of the essential omega 3 and 6 fatty acids. This is a much more natural food for you to consume, and due to the high chlorophyll content in the E3Live product, it helps to combat many diseases and supports the immune system in an amazing way. E3Live is said to be one of nature's most complete and nutrient-dense superfoods, and a great supplier of the fats that you need to support your body in order to have a long healthy life.

Feed Your Body with Oxygen – It's Called Exercise!

Every disease known to man can be helped and possibly successfully battled (am I allowed to say that?) by increasing circulation, body temperature, and adding oxygen. The body has two circulation systems, one for the lymphatic system, which helps to provide nutrients including oxygen and carries off wastes. The other system is for the blood, which is lucky enough to have a pump called your heart. Your lymphatic system needs your help in the form of exercise. It needs jigging about like a human shaker to get everything moving and stimulated. If the lymph does not circulate then the tissues suffocate by sitting in the stagnation of their own acidic waste products.

If your health is below par, try and gather whatever energy you can, get outside, and get moving. I hope that doesn't sound too harsh, but less than a third of the population exercises adequately, and I have seen first-hand that this not only affects your waistline, but your emotions, biochemistry, immune system, and rate of ageing. Stagnation and lack of movement can lead to disease. It has been proven over time that aerobic exercise, due to inhaling increased amounts of oxygen, will dramatically increase the pace of recovery for most patients who are suffering from a disease, let alone provide enormous benefits to those of you that are blessed with good health already. Resistance exercise such as weight-lifting, or using your own body weight, as in yoga, not only forms a healthy functional muscular structure, but also solidifies and strengthens the skeletal system. In both cases the positive effects are numerous, extending mental functionality and feelings of good mood.

If a person exercises, they will naturally have increased positivity and less tendency to procrastinate. Their self-esteem will be higher because they feel good in themselves and it can quickly change and improve your body shape. The strength that you gain makes you stand taller, have fewer aches and pains, and will enhance movement. Exercise also makes you feel sexier and more alive. It's so important in this age of busy lifestyles to help our bodies manage stress. We as humans are not meant to lead sedentary lifestyles. We are limiting the body so much, on a daily basis, that when some of us do eventually try to do things without the correct preparation, we end up getting injured … and so we give up. Joint operations on knees, shoulders, and hips are at an all-time high. I have a friend that has had over 13 operations on his knee, just to correct surgery. I am not for one moment knocking the amazing surgeons for the jobs they do. They improve people's quality of life every day and it's wonderful. What I am concerned with is the lack of knowledge and sporadic training that I see with many clients. They have great intentions, but the stop-start approach is dangerous as its doesn't build up the muscles well enough to be able to cope with the activity. Plus, if we are not getting the correct nutritional intake, and the body is challenged by malnutrition, it's a recipe for disaster.

Centuries ago we would be moving every day, farming, digging, sewing, baking, making … this offered us the full spectrum of aerobic and weightlifting exercise that is a prerequisite for health. Abnormal standing, leaning, sitting, and resting increased as the Industrial Revolution began in the nineteenth century. Many people started to migrate to cities and work situations began to change. Our world began to restrict the use of our bodies, making us weaker. Lack of body use, eating more processed foods and ready meals, gaining weight, and feeling depressed have paralysed the population, including the young.

I am at massive risk of sounding like a crazy old person here, but it breaks my heart when I see and hear of kids spending endless hours, days, months, years of their precious time playing sedentary computer games. It's criminal that they have no idea that they are being robbed of their childhood … their true imagination, the art of make-believe, and the lack of violence. I sincerely believe it is behind many of the mental health issues that we see amongst our young. Never before in my clinics have I seen so many depressed teenagers and young children. I know the pressure on them is enormous right now, and the pressure of obtaining good grades in exams is partly to blame. As is the endless pressure of celebrity 'perfect bodies' and social media, with its 'got to live up to that perfect life' existence. It's coming at them from all angles, so if you have children, you've got to play your part in helping to break this cycle.

It's not that they have to stop completely, or that they need to drop out of conforming to society. I love to watch a good film with my children and snuggle up on the sofa. We all spend a considerable amount of time on social media both for business and keeping up with friends, and my son plays Xbox from time to time. *But* … I always make sure that they are doing some form of exercise every day, even if it is just an hour's walk with our little dog. The basic fact is we all need to spend time outdoors. It's not just about going to the gym and working out in artificial lighting and air-conditioned rooms. I have worked in many hot climates over the last few years and I still can't believe how many people are deficient in vitamin D. They can live in one of the most sun-drenched places on the planet and are still deficient in the very vitamin they could get the most of. Why? Because many of them spend hours in air-conditioned homes, then get into their air-conditioned cars, and go to air-conditioned gyms. So they are not getting the chance to absorb this life-enhancing vitamin. And that is exactly what's happening to our children, and to us adults that work at office computers all day sitting on our butts.

We need to move! And shake it all about! When the body is not fuelled with oxygen and has no movement it gets stagnant, like a dirty old pond! You know, at first it looks clear and rich in health. Then, slowly, a build-up of algae starts to happen, the water becomes murky and toxic-looking, and before you know it not much can live in there. When your body is stagnant it is a prime environment for dis-ease to manifest! Yes dis-ease, meaning disharmony within our bodies. Things start to go wrong, you feel pain or discomfort somewhere, you feel lifeless and lethargic, and you don't want to do much.

If I were to tell you there is a drug I can give you that is free, and will help prevent sleep disorders, memory malfunctions, heart disease, blood pressure, infertility, erectile dysfunction, cancers, obesity, diabetes, fatigue, depression, and so much more, what would you do? Take it? Yes of course you would. This drug is called exercise! We spend billions of dollars and pounds worldwide on health care dispensing medicines, running tests, researching illnesses. What about this simple prevention method? All you need is a starting base of 30 mins per day five times a week. I know for some people that may be a lot, but in the grand scheme of hours in your day it's nothing. It has to be a priority because exercise can help prevent, alleviate, or treat almost every disease state. You also need to be doing at least one and a half hours of weight training per week as a minimum. And if you are over 40 you need to be stretching for at least 30 minutes every single day! Without exception.

Take depression as a classic example. If you are exercising it produces changes in the part of the brain that regulates stress and anxiety. It also increases brain sensitivity for the hormones serotonin and norepinephrine, which relieves feelings of low mood. It increases the production of endorphins, which are known to help produce positive feelings and reduce the perception of pain. In the film *Legally Blonde*, when Elle is becoming a lawyer and is trying to prove her client's innocence, she says, in some of the most memorable lines in the movie: 'Exercise gives you endorphins. Endorphins make you happy and happy people just don't shoot their husbands.' Classic! Hilarious, but many a true word is spoken in jest!

Weight loss is easier when reducing calorie intake because it increases your metabolic rate which in turn burns more calories, helping you to lose weight. Combining aerobic exercise or cardiovascular exercise with resistance training, such a push-ups, sit-ups, or weights can maximize fat loss and help tone and strengthen muscles. Having better

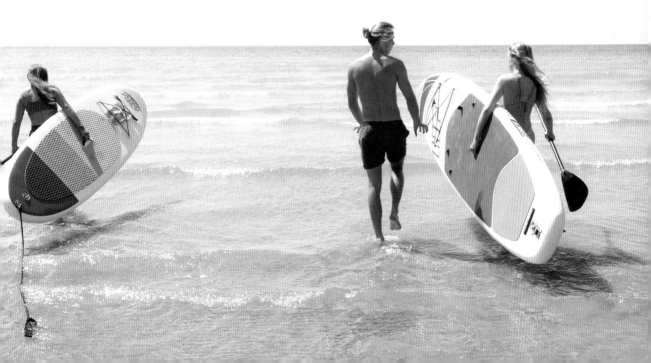

conditioned muscles gives you stronger bones, preventing osteoporosis. It gives you a better posture, which allows the body to flow properly! Not stagnate. Exercise can significantly improve energy levels, even for those suffering from fatigue. It reduces your risk of chronic disease and it can help you look amazing. Regular moderate exercise can also increase your body's production of natural antioxidants which help protect your cells. It helps stimulate blood flow, improves brain function, and protects memory and thinking skills. To begin with it increases your heart rate, which promotes the flow of blood and oxygen to your brain. Then it stimulates the production of hormones, that can enhance the growth of brain cells and causes the hippocampus (a part of the brain that's vital for memory and learning) to grow in size.

It has also been shown to reduce changes in the brain that can cause Alzheimer's and schizophrenia. When you exercise your sleep quality is better because the energy depletion that occurs during exercise stimulates recuperative processes during sleep. Just 150 minutes of light to moderate exercise per week has been shown to provide up to a 65 per cent improvement in sleep quality. For many years the recommendation for chronic pain was rest. Now, exercise is being used to help control pain such as a lower back pain, fibromyalgia, and soft tissue disorders, partly because it can raise pain tolerance and reduce pain perception.

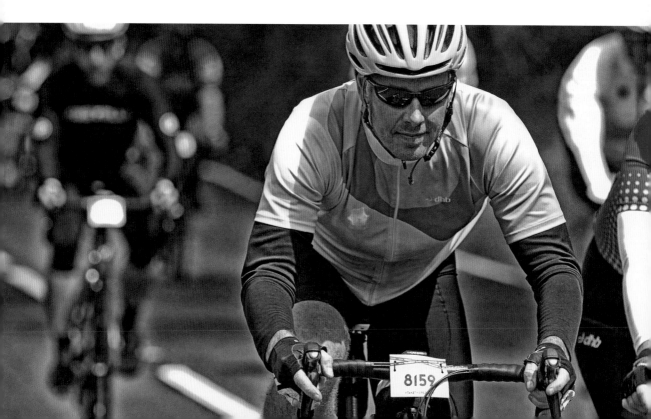

Engaging in regular exercise has a benefit that I don't think any of us will argue with. Due to strengthening the cardiovascular system, improving blood circulation, toning muscles, and enhancing flexibility, it can not only improve your sexual performance and sexual pleasure, it increases the frequency of sexual activity. So what's not to love?

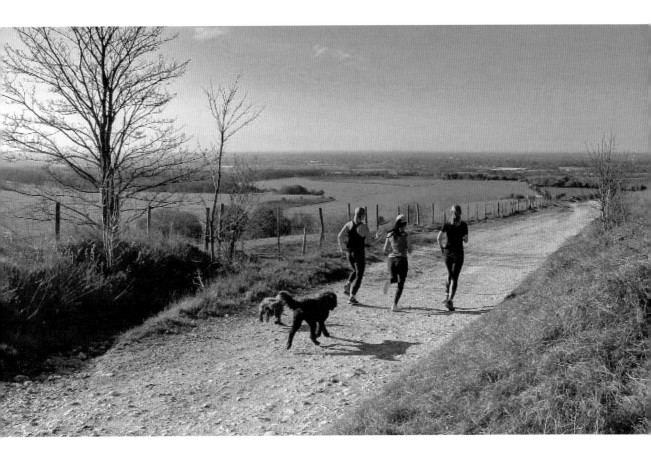

The bottom line is this: exercising regularly is one of the best things you can do for your health. Within days of starting to exercise you will notice a difference in how you feel. Work out a way that you can incorporate regular exercise into your daily routine and try to create a plan that is realistic for you. Having an exercise buddy (I have three girlfriends that I regularly run with – without them I would stay in bed on dark winter days, but they would literally freak out! Having them in my ear on days when I feel like I just want an extra 10 minutes in bed is beyond brilliant. I am grateful for them every day as we spur each other on, not only to get to the starting point of the run, but to do more mileage, different routes, longer runs, etc.). If you have someone to be accountable to if you don't turn up, it's a far greater incentive than being a lone wolf. On the other hand, if you have a crazy busy job, and exercise is your solitude, then it's probably best you work out alone.

You need to work out what is better suited to your lifestyle and what your own needs are. The other key factor to regular successful exercising is making it a routine … part of your daily life. I always do my cardio workout first thing in the morning. I like it because I feel it sets me up mentally for the day and makes me feel vibrant and energized. Some people can't do it until later in the day because of time restraints, but whatever you do, try to get your regular routine going so each week you know where you are and when you are going to be doing it. Your body will begin to crave more, because it feels soooo good! Last, but by no means least, make it fun. The more you love it, the more likely you are to do it. If you love music and dancing, then go for that. Whatever takes your fancy. Experiment with different exercises and see what brings you the most joy and happiness and embrace it. It could just save your life.

Mindful Exercise

Resting and creating peace with meditation and yoga can have a profound and transformative effect on your health. I think a lot of us, and I included myself in this category for many years, think that if we are charging around and getting a million things achieved in one day, we are completely brilliant. Well, yes, on one hand we are, but on the other hand it's going to have consequences eventually. Resting the mind and the body is just as important as the food that we eat, the exercise we take part in, and the company we surround ourselves with.

It also makes me wonder why most of the classes I attend are female dominated. Men that do yoga have amazing physiques, and personally I don't think there is anything sexier than seeing a man lay down his tools after work, get a pair of sweatpants on, and perform yoga for two hours. There are plenty of macho guys that are taking up yoga as a regular practice, because they can see and feel the benefits this amazing sport can bring them, but if you are a guy reading this book and you haven't given yoga a chance, go check it out, because if you think it's just for girls, it really isn't. The physique you can get from regular yoga is incredible and powerful. Using your own body weight to create muscle is probably the safest and most effective way to tone up, but the peace that it creates in your headspace is the bit that I want to focus on. Things are changing rapidly in society, and certain practices are becoming more mainstream and acceptable.

Teaching yoga in schools, for example, is becoming more widely accepted; and in prisons for both inmates and officers it's producing incredibly positive results. Can you imagine a world where everyone had to start their day off with an hour of yoga? I believe that if it was mandatory to go to work and be forced to take part in 30 minutes of stretching and weight-bearing yoga and half an hour of guided meditation on lifting your own vibration and positivity the world would be an extremely different place to live. So, I get down on my knees and beg you, please just have a go. Maybe try at least four different types of yoga before you settle on a class that you love. There are many different styles and types, and some may suit you more than others.

Hatha yoga: this is a classic approach to breathing and exercise and is a great entry point for beginners.

Iyengar yoga: this focuses on alignment as well as detailed practice movements whilst controlling the breath. It's great for people with injuries who need to work slowly and methodically.

Kundalini yoga: this is equal parts spiritual and physical. It's about releasing the kundalini energy said to be trapped in the body. These classes are perhaps more intense and can involve quite a bit of chanting, mantras, and meditation. I personally love kundalini and feel completely invigorated and peaceful after a class. I have taken my children to all varieties of yoga and this was to be honest the one they struggled with the most, getting a complete fit of the giggles when asked to pant like a dog for five minutes and snore like an old man for two. It was a small disaster, but luckily, I know the very lovely instructor well and she was forgiving of the outbursts. Needless to say, they didn't come back to these classes with me, although they do take part in hatha, and it's helping exam pressure enormously. Maybe when they are adults, they might go back to the more spiritual type. Let's see!

Ashtanga yoga: this involves physically demanding sequences of postures, and may be not quite so suited to beginners, but great for you fit bods who require more demanding stuff!

Vinyasa yoga: this is perhaps the most athletic style. It was adapted from ashtanga in the 1980s and in classes the movement is coordinated with your breath and movement to flow from one pose to another. Many types of yoga can also be considered vinyasa flows, such as ashtanga, power yoga, and prana and the styles can vary depending upon the teacher. I have been to many classes that combine styles and it's great.

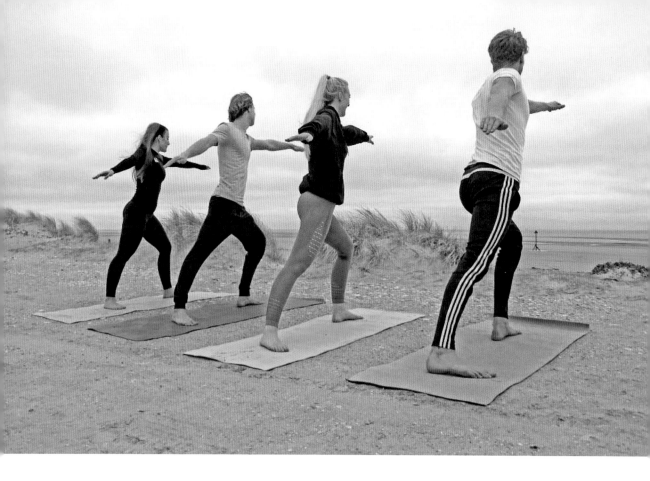

Bikram yoga: this is better known now as hot yoga. It features a sequence of set poses in a sauna/hot-style room of about 105 degrees and 40% humidity. The first time I attended a hot yoga class I went with my sports shorts on and a t-shirt and felt completely overdressed. I was greeted in the yoga room by a man with only a G-string on and girls in bikinis. Not that I have any issues with nudity at all, it was just a little unexpected on my first experience. However, when doing a downward dog I was standing directly behind the aforementioned gentleman in the tiny briefs, his left testicle popped out of his pants and remained there for the entire rest of the class. I did wonder momentarily if this was the class for me.

Yin yoga: this is a slow-paced style with seated postures that are held for long periods of time. This is a great class for beginners. It's also a meditative yoga, helping the participant to find inner peace.

Restorative yoga: this focuses on chilling out after the day and relaxing your mind. It focuses mostly on body relaxation and is such a wonderful thing to do at the end of a busy week.

Prenatal yoga: this is carefully adapted for 'mums to be' and is for all trimesters throughout the pregnancy. It's great for pelvic floor work, and fantastic for breathing and bonding with the growing baby. It can also help mothers prepare for the delivery and labour.

Anusara yoga: this is a modern-day version of hatha yoga and focuses on alignment, with more focus on the mind, body, and heart connection.

Jivamukti yoga: this is mainly vinyasa flow-style classes with spiritual teachings. Starting with a series of chants followed by a series of poses that align with the five tenets of jivamukti yoga and philosophy. This style emphasizes its connection to the earth as a living being.

You know some nights when you get home and there are so many other things to do apart from yoga and you force yourself to turn around and go? What if that turned out to be the best hour and a half of your day and worth every second you are there for your physical, emotional, and mental well-being. The times you are resistant to going are when you probably need it the most! As you can see, there are many types, and probably more still as I don't profess to be the expert on yoga, so do your research and find out what classes are near you and if you haven't already taken part in a class, go and see what it's all about. There are so many health benefits in incorporating this into your life, it's almost insane not to.

As we get older, flexibility becomes more important. There was a lady on the news recently that starting practising yoga at the age of 90! And now at the age of 99 she is still going strong and is more flexible than ever. This is a great lesson showing quite clearly that it's never too late to start anything. When you first begin you may feel completely immobile and not be able to go anywhere near touching your toes, but stick with it and you will notice how amazingly reactive your body is. Your aches and pains start to disappear because your tight, stiff hips, once loosened, will improve your knee and ankle joints, as well as improving alignment for your back, arms, legs, and entire posture. When you build strength in your body, it can help prevent conditions such as arthritis, heal injuries, and improve your balance, which is crucial at any age. Taking your joints through a full range of movement helps them to receive fresh nutrients, keeping them healthy. That's why putting yoga and amazing nutrition together could add another 10 years to your life. Stronger muscles create stronger bones – that's a fact. This is beneficial for every bone in your body but particularly your spine, helping to protect you from osteoporosis, back problems, and pain related to weakness.

Remember I mentioned before, getting your blood flowing properly is key to sustaining great health? Well, yoga is perfect for pumping more oxygen into your cells and boosting haemoglobin and red blood cells. It thins the blood by making platelets less sticky (I always refer to it as tomato ketchup blood). This can lead to a decrease in heart attacks and strokes since blood clots are often the cause of these killers. Because your circulation is stimulated it helps clean and drain your precious lymphatic system, keeping you free from toxins, and making you more resilient when it comes to fighting infection. It can protect you massively and destroys cancerous cells, due to the nutrients and goodness being delivered. Remind yourself often that it's almost impossible for disease to manifest in a nutrient-rich, relaxed, and oxygenated body.

Improving the strength of your heart is an added bonus from yoga, as well as helping lift feelings of low mood and depression. Yoga also contributes to balancing your blood pressure and regulating your exhausted adrenal glands due to its ability to lower cortisol levels in your body. The overproduction of cortisol is poisonous to you and we need to get rid of it in excess. But better still, yoga increases your levels of serotonin which help you feel happy, and this has a knock-on effect, creating the cycle for better sleep, and in turn helping to maintain a healthy nervous system. As yoga teaches you to relax, your whole system will thank you for it. When you slow your breath and concentrate only on being present in this very moment, you immediately shift the balance from your sympathetic nervous system (the fight or flight, ready-to-kill stage) to the parasympathetic nervous system, which is calming and restorative to all organs in the body, including your intestines and reproductive organs.

It's a fact: meditation can literally change your life. If you wake up at 4 a.m. and your mind is buzzing with things you need to do the next day then you need to listen up. Or if you lack confidence, get anxious, feel overwhelmed, or have no direction in life … then where have you been? A ton of celebrities speak openly about their daily meditation and how it rewires the brain. Celebrities such as Michael Jordan, Oprah Winfrey, Paul McCartney, Richard Branson, Eva Mendez, Arnold Schwarzenegger and many more have all been vocal about how effective this practice is and how much it has helped in their lives. Whether it's part of your yoga session, or a separate practice, find time to fit it into your day. Personally, I love guided meditation on subjects such as love, success, creating abundance, happiness, peace, tranquillity and calming the mind. If you don't want to go to a class, then go on YouTube. There are so many self-help guided meditations that you can do night after night, or first thing in the morning, or preferably both if you can.

I couldn't believe the mind-blowing effect that meditation had on me when I first started. It's mighty powerful and changes your whole outlook on everything. Don't worry, you're not going to become some ganja-smoking hippie because you started to meditate (and if you do that's your choice!). And it's not going to turn you into a bore … far from it my gorgeousnesses! You are going to become quite the Adonis or the Aphrodite! The most significant thing I have noticed since meditating is the ability to manifest what I really want. So, you end up attracting the right people, have space in your head for more creativity, draw strength to leave situations that no longer serve you, and gain knowledge and brain power like never before. It allows you to draw away from certain topics or people that feel negative, make better decisions, have more patience, more tolerance, more laughter, richer relationships, and generally more time. The list goes on and on and there is real science behind it for those sceptics out there. Meditation really does increase your psychological functioning and in the process improves your sense of well-being. According to studies, meditation, yoga, and tai chi have all been found to have such therapeutic effects when practised regularly that they can increase healthy lifespan by years. Meditation can also connect you better to others, and I am not just talking about your loved ones, although this is a wonderful part of your meditation experience. Relationships improve throughout. Work colleagues, gym buddies, friends, associates, the stranger walking their dog, the dustman emptying your rubbish, the shop assistant who serves you.

Meditation can reach areas of your brain that are associated with mental processing and empathy and increases your sense of social connectedness and ability to relate to others. It improves your ability to read how others are feeling, due to your increased focus, emotional stability, and sense of calm. When we strengthen the connection between the heart and the mind with regular practice, we allow ourselves to feel the beauty, joy, and wonder of the world that surrounds us. The mind is more powerful than perhaps we could ever know. One of the most amazing benefits of meditation is that it has the capability to reduce mental and physical pain. Yes that's correct! Imagine, if it can do such things, how effective it can be when dealing with anxiety, stress, and depression.

Again, I am not criticizing anyone in any way, whether medical or non-medical, but if a person goes to visit a doctor saying they are depressed, why are they not prescribed an immediate six sessions of meditation to see how they feel? Instead we have people roaming our planet so numb, so zoned out from 'feeling' anything at all they cannot possibly know what's real and what's not. Are they happy, are they sad? Can they cry when they need to? Laugh if they feel like it? I have seen clients that literally feel nothing, and giving a person other options before a lifetime of drugs must surely be a priority? If a person is given six sessions of meditation, they might just see the world in a completely different light and want to continue on that path and bring it into their daily lives forever.

The other thing is the cleaner you are living (less junk and processed food, alcohol, drugs, etc.), the more profound an effect these things are going to have on you. But you have to start somewhere: it's another 'chicken or egg' situation! If you start cleaning up your diet first, you will be more inspired to get mentally strong and create the pathway in order to implement other changes. If you start meditation or yoga first, you will create a better environment and calmer brain in order to process what you need in relation to nutrition. They all lead back to each other eventually and when you start aligning in this way, it feels truly magical and you feel very much in control of your destiny.

I believe meditation can create radical changes that reduce anxiety-related disorders and also increase your stress resilience. When we are able to switch off the fight or flight response and trigger relaxation on a regular basis, we are training our bodies – just as we do in the gym when we want to build muscle – to learn how to quickly stabilize and rapidly recover from the impact of stress. So instead of being in that cortisol-releasing state of heightened anxiousness, we can easily move into the calm zone when facing challenges or life demands. In the same way meditation can induce feelings of calm it can also evoke positive emotions because of the reduction of stress. We are then able to become much more connected to ourselves, feeling more confident and happier in everyday situations.

Meditating also has a dramatic effect on the prefrontal cortex and how much it gets stimulated. This part of the brain involves problem-solving, concentration, focus, and emotional intelligence. We become less reactive, less defensive, and effortlessly balanced more of the time. If you require more brain volume – in other words, you need to retain more information because you are learning something new, or studying for exams, or learning lines for a new role in a movie, whatever it is – when you meditate regularly you increase the capacity to retain information, therefore you are learning better and more efficiently. This information should be part of every school curriculum from the age of five and should be regarded as normal learning, just as good nutrition should be taught.

When my children were little, I set up a company called Fit Kids. I had loads of friends that wanted to exercise but didn't have time because they were looking after their little ones. It was a boot camp that took parents off one way and children the other. There was an hour of exercise and then half an hour nutrition teaching and smoothie making and experimenting at the end. It was so much fun, and everyone loved it. The children were eating spinach and all sorts of other fruits and vegetables. Yoga, meditation, and good healthy food is very interesting if it is presented that way, and everyone, including the children, becomes hungry for the knowledge once it's exposed to them. Education is everything.

From a physical perspective, meditation is very powerful when it comes to your immune system. I believe it helps it to be strong, cutting off the routes by which you catch a cold or get sick, especially when it comes to more serious diseases. It regulates blood pressure and heart rate and significantly slows down the ageing process. So don't book your facelift just yet, just meditate more because it triggers the release of melatonin and DHEA and decreases cortisol which impacts on how you age. Remember, it's never too late to start. If you want things to change, start making things happen and start now. Your fabulous cells are there, ready and waiting! They are renewing all the time, so anything is possible.

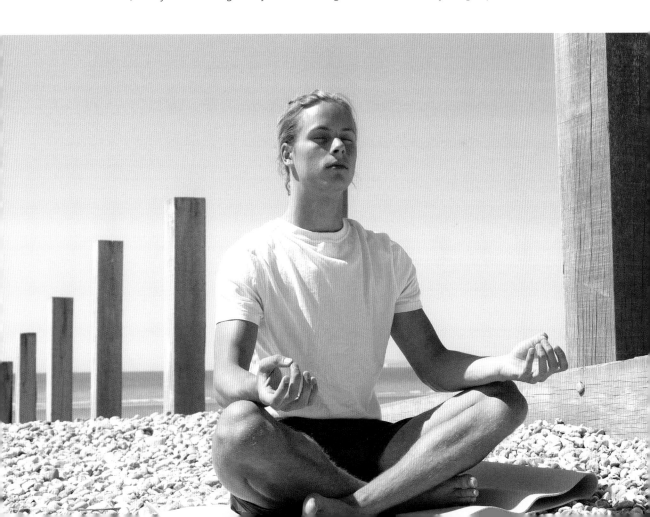

If you are just starting out with meditation, I would suggest you begin with anything from 5–10 minutes per day, at least five times a week. Within a two-week period, you will start to notice significant differences and shifts in how you feel. When I first started, I honestly noticed shifts within two days.

What do you have to lose?

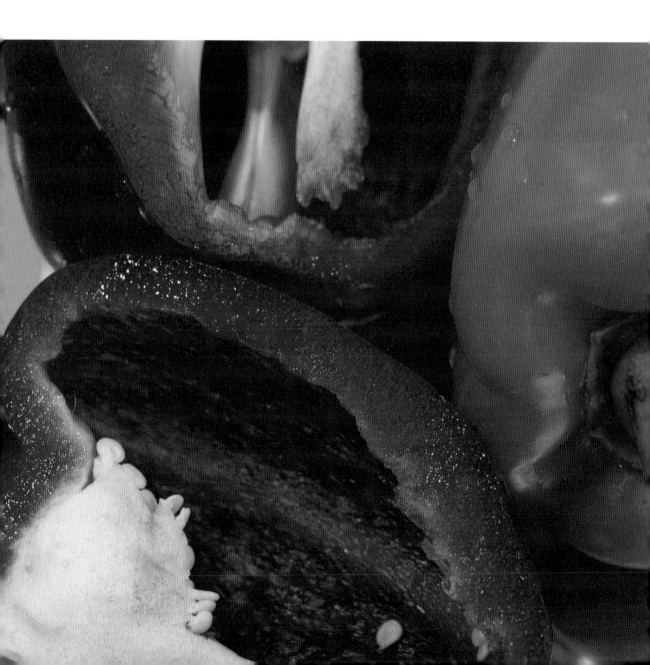

CHAPTER 5

LET'S STOP THE PREMATURE DYING

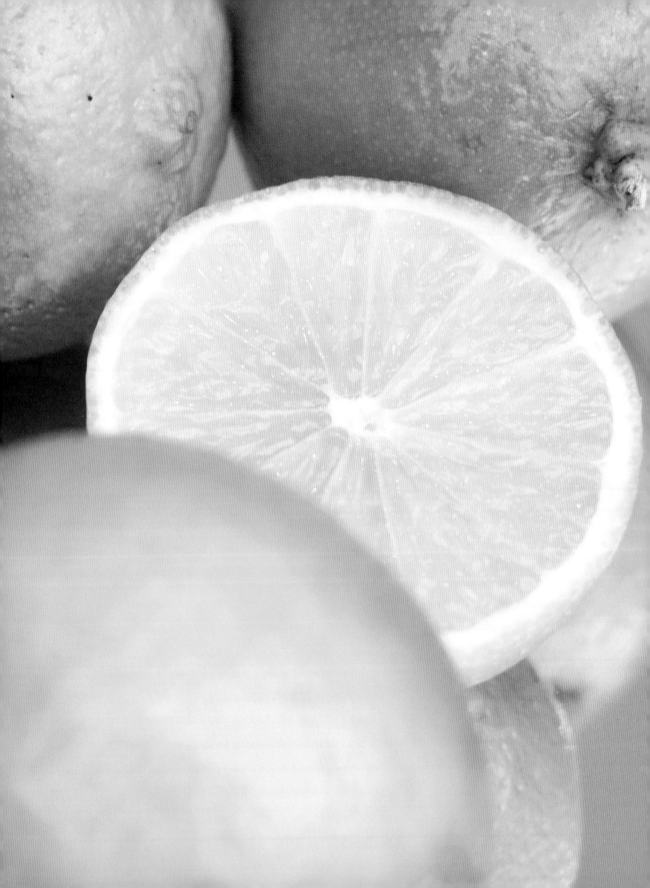

What do you want out of life? To climb the ladder of success? To run your own company? Or perhaps you wish to free up your time so you can travel more? Or you want to be a fantastic parent or grandparent? Or you want to go to university to study? Or become a musician or movie star and globe-trot all over the world making your fortune. It doesn't really matter what you want to do, or how you want to live your life. The bottom line is that having good health enables you to do more of the things that you want without worry or concern. Health challenges may cause setbacks for you, so why not get on the right path in order to achieve vibrant health right now?

We live in an age where millions of pounds and dollars are spent on medical research each year. There have been huge medical advances in understanding disease, but what about curing it? More and more people in the world are getting sick. Our life expectancy is higher, and people are living with disease, but what about curing, or stopping the disease from manifesting in the first place? Research into whole living foods suggests that pretty much every organ in the body can be healed over time. The stomach lining, for example, when given the correct foods, smoothies, juices, superfoods, and herbs, can repair itself in as little as five days. The intestinal lining takes as little as seven days. Isn't that insane when you think of the number of people you and I know that have stomach issues? Colitis, irritable bowel syndrome, inflammation of the gut, polyps, leaky gut, acid reflux, ulcers, not to mention digestive cancers. The list is endless, and the amount of medication that is used to try and control these diseases is vast.

Some cancers have a genetic component, but often it's the lifestyle choices that pull the trigger. Digestive-related cancers are more likely to be the result of poor lifestyle choices, and that is something you can help to prevent. Disease does not just pop up overnight. It may take years for things to manifest, cells to change, so don't ignore symptoms, do something about them. Food is our greatest exposure to the outside environment, and if you think that the food you eat has nothing to do with the way you feel every day then think again.

Your intestines, if taken out of your body, could cover the surface of a tennis court. If you think shoving processed fast food down your gullet a good idea, then think again. The 'beige' food, as I call it, can get stuck, be horrendously acidic, high in fats and sugar, and do absolutely nothing for you nutritionally whatsoever. It's a traffic jam waiting to happen, and it keeps getting piled in day after day. Then you get blobs of cellulite and wonder where it has suddenly come from. A little belly grows and grows until one day you are three clothes sizes bigger and you have no idea how that happened. Excessive weight can potentially increase the chance of cancer growth, diabetes, heart disease, and tumours. A life of processed foods, stimulants, dark cold climates, and disharmonious relationships are the gateway to disease and death! Be real with yourself. It's no crime to get caught up in this way of living. Lots of people comfort eat, right? And in my opinion that is the very reason people are dying young, suffering more from depression, are more mentally exhausted than ever, angrier and more frustrated, in constant pain, and feeling generally and utterly yuck.

Colon and rectal cancers are amongst the most commonly diagnosed cancers in the Western world. But they are rare in other parts of the world such as India. Why is this? Is it their food intake? Could it be that as a country they eat very little meat compared to us? They consume legumes, beans, split peas, chickpeas, and lentils on a daily basis and a shedload of dark green leafy vegetables which are packed with phytates (an incredible powerful anti-cancer fighting compound). Also think about the amount of spices and herbs that they use in their cooking. Turmeric is a key ingredient for them, and this is an anti-inflammatory spice we could all benefit from on a daily basis, with life-saving cancer-fighting properties. They are also one of the largest producers of fruits and vegetables, so they have access to fresh produce every day.

Take pancreatic cancer as another example. On average, only 6% of patients survive more than five years after diagnosis. There have been connections made between this disease and the consumption of fat from animal sources for many years now.

So surely prevention must be far better than cure? If you understood that every single substance that passes through your lips has a profound effect on your body in one way or another, wouldn't this encourage you to make different choices? No such link has ever been found when consuming the majority of plant-based foods. And don't think this just means red meats either. I often meet people who say they don't eat meat, and what they actually mean is they don't eat red meat, but they do consume chicken, duck, pork, etc. An study investigating links between cancer and nutrition (the European Prospective Investigation into Cancer and Nutrition (EPIC)), which followed 477,000 people over a 10-year period, found a 72% increased risk of pancreatic cancer for every 50 grams of poultry consumed daily. We need a plant-based diet in order to avoid this.

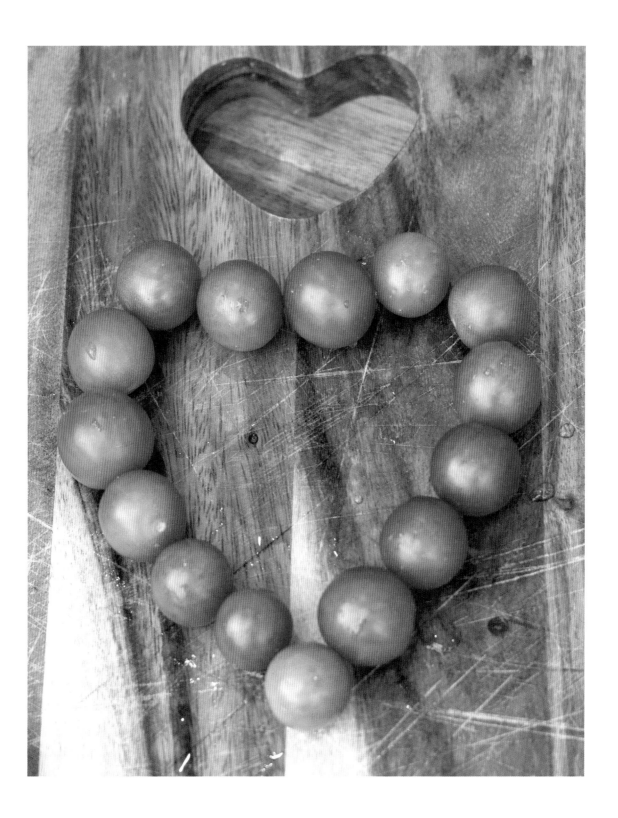

Heart Disease

Up there with the number one killers in the world is heart disease. It kills an estimated 17.9 million people worldwide and dietary choices can mean the difference between life or death. Heart disease is responsible for one in three deaths for both males and females over the age of 50. If you have ever read Dr Campbell's best-selling book *The China Study*, then you may just think twice about the amount of meat you consume. If at all … ever again! He examined the dietary habits and mortality rates of several hundreds of thousands of people in rural China. Their diets were much more plant-based, and the study concluded that they suffered a hundred times fewer heart attacks compared to the average American of the same age. It was even suggested that heart disease may start in the womb if your mother had high cholesterol. Eating a standard Western diet can mean that the plaque build-up is there without any symptoms. But if it was spotted in time, and the person was put on a plant-based diet, and a few other healthy lifestyle changes were made, they could in fact reverse their disease and avoid surgery or further symptoms such as pain and shortness of breath.

Strokes

During a stroke the blood flow to the brain is cut off, depriving it of oxygen, causing brain cells to die, making it a medical emergency. It can be caused by narrowing or blockages of the arteries. These blockages are often caused by blood clots, which can have serious consequences. Depending on which area of the brain is damaged, it can have a massive impact on the severity of the condition and recovery from it. A major stroke can mean paralysis, losing the ability to speak, coma, or death. Mild strokes can mean weakness in a limb, vision problems in one or both eyes, dizziness and loss of balance, or slurring words and confusion. Again, a plant-based diet and regular exercise may help to reduce your odds of having a stroke. If you knew the simple things you could do daily that would help prevent such potentially life-changing events it could be so easy to achieve. Just 7 grams per day of fibre, (only found in fruits or vegetables), such as one cup of raspberries, is associated with a 7% risk reduction. Or increasing your potassium intake with half a cup of green beans, you can reduce your risk by 21%. So simple, yet so effective.

Diabetes

This disease has been referred to as the 'Black Death' of the twenty-first century. It's not just the disease itself that can be life-restricting and difficult to cope with, but all the issues that go with it. Diabetes can cause loss of vision, kidney failure, lower extremity amputations, heart attacks, and strokes, and it is responsible for an estimated 1.5 million deaths each year worldwide. There are two types of diabetes, type 1 and type 2. Both types are chronic diseases that affect the way your body regulates blood sugar and glucose. Glucose is the fuel that is needed to feed your cells, but to gain entrance to your cells it needs a key. That key is called insulin. If you have type 1 diabetes you don't produce insulin because your pancreas no longer makes it, so you have to inject it to control your blood glucose levels. People with type 2 diabetes don't respond to insulin as well as they should and later in the course of the disease often don't make enough insulin. Blood sugar control is the most important element in keeping this disease under control. Prescription medication in the form of pills is prescribed for this condition and the right lifestyle choices are essential.

Insulin is a vital hormone that shuttles glucose (blood sugar) into our cells, preventing dangerous levels from accumulating in the blood. Insulin resistance is primarily caused by fatty build-up inside our muscle cells. This can come from too much fat in our bodies, or excess fat from our food. Either way around 90% of people who develop diabetes are overweight. Eating a plant-based diet can help you not only to shed the pounds but restore the body's ability to heal. In many studies in the USA and Canada people who reduced, or cut out completely, fish, dairy, eggs, and meat appear to have a 78% reduced risk of diabetes. Adding beans to your diet has been found to improve blood sugar markers and help with weight loss as much as calorie cutting and portion control. There is a slight warning here: because your body is so remarkable, if you start to heal too quickly and are on prescription medication for your condition, you may need some medical supervision as your blood pressure and blood sugars can drop too low too quickly.

Liver Disease

This is often associated with high alcohol consumption or drug use, but, alarmingly, fatty liver disease from certain food choices is quietly creeping in as the most common form of chronic liver disease. In other words, all the fats and sugars in the foods that we are eating are clogging up that precious organ we rely on so heavily to keep us well. Liver disease accounts for approximately 2 million deaths worldwide, 1 million due to complications of cirrhosis and 1 million due to hepatitis and hepatocellular carcinomas (the most common type of liver cancer). Alcoholic fatty liver disease begins with the build-up of fats in the liver. This leads to inflammation and scarring and cirrhosis. And it is said that drinking even one can of fizzy drink daily can raise your odds of fatty liver disease substantially. I know families that consume large amounts of fizzy drinks at every mealtime. Think of the damage they are doing, when you could just have a glass of health-enhancing hydration called H2O! A plant-based diet can help cleanse the liver and give your body the nutrients it needs and also eating oatmeal has been found to significantly improve liver function amongst both men and women and to help with weight loss too. People that also consume whole wheat, brown rice, and more fruits and vegetables can help avoid developing such disease.

Kidneys

Healthy kidneys filter about half a cup of blood every minute, removing waste and extra water to make urine. If your kidneys are not working properly it can lead to serious issues such as shortness of breath, abnormal heart rhythms, weakness, and confusion due to the metabolic waste products that accumulate in the blood and will essentially poison you to death. In certain people that are already extremely stressed, with their poor adrenal glands at bursting point, drinking too much caffeine can have a detrimental effect. Caffeine causes a short but sudden increase in blood pressure, which can also increase the rate of decline in the way the kidneys function. Not to mention the many hidden chemicals that may be added to your favourite fizzy drink too. This all contributes to extra toxicity for the body to deal with and your beautiful little kidney beans that are desperately trying to extract waste from your blood, balance your body fluids, form urine, and produce hormones that help regulate blood pressure and control calcium metabolism, struggle to cope. An estimated 7.1 million people worldwide die of kidney disease and it is said that animal protein can trigger inflammatory reactions to your kidneys, causing them to be less efficient as you age. A plant-based diet with plenty of hydration and exercise is said to help preserve and nurture these organs that we take for granted. Once your kidneys reach a certain level of damage a transplant is needed, and the risks associated with this are high. Taking care of your kidneys is essential.

Lungs

Lung cancer is the leading type of cancer in both men and women worldwide and is responsible for 29% of cancer deaths, more than cancer of the breast, colon, and prostate combined. Chronic obstructive pulmonary disease (COPD) and asthma collectively kill 296,000 Americans every year. A plant-based diet is said to significantly reduce all three. Asthma can be helped simply by adding a few more servings of fruit and vegetables into your diet and research done on this topic indicates that this can cut asthmatic conditions significantly. Never think that eating better is not going to help. Obviously preventing lung cancer by giving up smoking is advisable, but that is not always the cause. Did you know that a single stalk of broccoli per day can boost activity of detoxifying enzymes in the liver, helping to prevent lung cancer due to the effect on the DNA damage at a cellular level? Emphysema is another condition that makes it hard to breathe, and the disease gradually worsens over time. Increasing your daily servings of fruit and vegetables can lower the risks by over 24%.

Blood Cancers

People that consume a more plant-based diet are less likely to develop all forms of cancer, but this has the most effect on blood cancers such as leukaemia, lymphoma, and multiple myeloma. These can be referred to as the liquid tumours since the cancer cells often circulate throughout the body rather than being concentrated in a solid mass. The Mayo Clinic has conducted many studies and suggest that eating broccoli or other cruciferous vegetables can be associated with a lower risk of non-Hodgkin's lymphoma. Plus, people that ate three or more servings of green leafy vegetables per week appeared to have only half the risk of developing blood cancers. This protection must surely be due to the amount of antioxidants found in plant-based foods. Do not confuse this with supplements. As I have said many times it's much better to eat as nature intended.

Breast Cancer

In relation to this cancer, the food we eat is especially important. Postmenopausal women who eat grilled, barbecued, or smoked meats over their lifetime are at as much as a 47% higher risk of getting this disease. Eating in the same way as you do to help prevent heart disease is just as beneficial for you in the prevention of breast cancer, since this keeps your cholesterol levels under control. A high fibre diet is also associated with lowering your risks. Alcohol has also been associated with increasing your risk because of how much it interferes with oestrogen levels.

To help prevent breast cancer in both men and women, it's important to recognize the link between elevated hormones and ill health. Only 5% of breast cancers are directly related to genetics, but lifestyle choices can trigger them. So, an easy tip would be to stack up the seeds, such as flax, pumpkin, sunflower and sesame. They all help balance hormones. Eat plenty of vegetables every day. That's why I love smoothies as they allow you to get a larger quantity of vegetables and superfoods in one go! Add kale, broccoli, cauliflower, cabbage, and even start sprouting the seeds of your favourite life-enhancing vegetables (see more about this in Chapter 13).

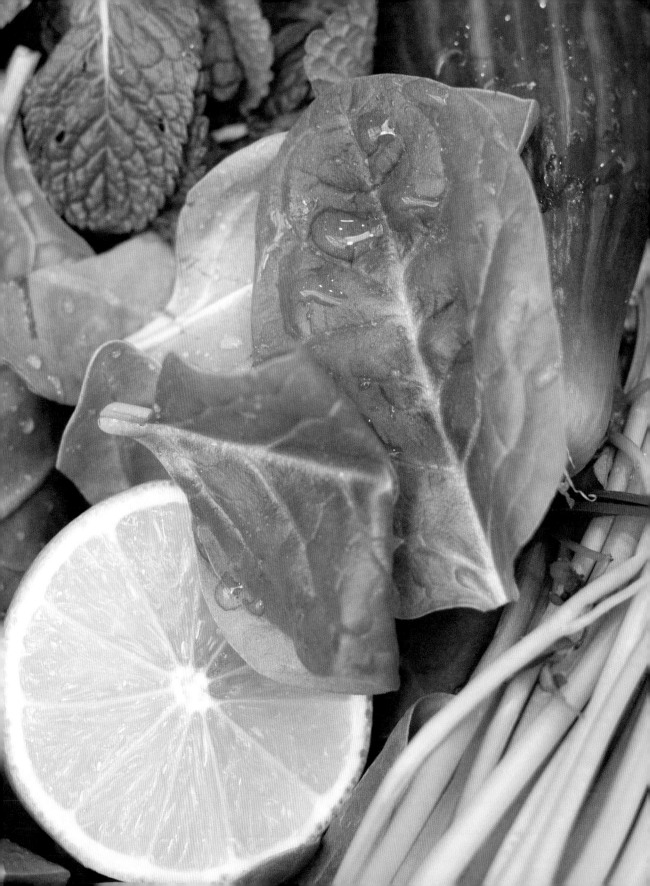

Add olive oil into your diet and take B vitamins that contain folate rather than folic acid (which is synthetic). Do not buy foods that are fortified with vitamins, such as breakfast cereals and bread. I know this is confusing because folate is vital to our overall health, but women taking more than 400mcg a day are at higher risk of breast cancers. Take the nutrients you need from your foods and superfoods, not man-made substances. Put a rainbow of colours on your plate every day. Tomatoes, for example, have positive impacts on the body as they help regulate hormones and fat and sugar metabolism. Looking after your liver will also help with hormone-related cancers. Minimize your intake of alcohol, sugars, and processed trans fats as they put a burden on the liver and upset your digestion. This could increase candida in your gut (an overgrowth of yeast that thrives on sugar) which can add stress to your immune system and which will certainly not help you to fight against cancer cells.

Prostate Cancer

One in nine men will be diagnosed with prostate cancer so it is more common than you think. The prostate is usually the size and shape of a walnut and grows bigger as you get older. It sits underneath the bladder and surrounds the urethra, which is the tube men urinate and ejaculate from. Its main job is to make semen, the fluid that carries sperm. High animal consumption and bad dietary choices can contribute to the manifestation of this disease, dairy being the most consistently associated with risk. What you need to do to prevent – or help if you already have this disease – is to stop the progression by simply adding more plant-based fruits and vegetables, such as carrots, tomatoes, broccoli, cauliflower, kale, pomegranates, grapes, grapefruit, oranges, lemons, limes, avocados, peppers, apples, berries, whole grains, and beans into your daily regime. Green tea has been particularly associated with both reduction and prevention due to the polyphenols and flavonoids it contains, both of which are very strong antioxidants. Tea is also the best source of catechins which are being studied for their anti-cancer properties.

Parkinson's Disease

This is caused by loss of nerve cells in the part of the brain called the substantia nigra, which means that the part of the brain controlling movement can't work as well as normal, causing movements to be slow. The loss of nerve cells is a slow process and it is still not completely certain what causes this disease although there are many different schools of thought. One is that head injuries can cause inflammation in the brain, leading to cell change which could result in structural changes contributing to the onset of Parkinson's. In a patient with this disease the brain cells that produce a chemical called dopamine begin to die off. Dopamine is important for the control of muscle movement and that is why patients have tremors, slowed movement, and stiffness. However, there is also a theory that brain damage can be caused by exposure to pollutants and toxic heavy metals that build up in the food supply. For example, the number one source of mercury is seafood, including tuna. Arsenic has been found in poultry and tuna, and lead is found in dairy products. Basically, the highest contamination of toxic chemicals has been found in fish, fish oils, eggs, dairy, and meats. The lowest combination was found at the bottom of the food chain, in plants. Those who base their diets around plants and wholefoods have significant lower levels of toxins, lowering their chances of developing this disease.

Infections

We live and breathe alongside thousands of potentially harmful bacteria. If we stopped to think about it, we would be scared to take a breath. Not only do we have pollutants outside in the streets, from traffic, factories, etc., but also in our very own homes: cleaning products, fabrics, protective chemicals on carpets, floors, sofas, etc. So how do we keep safe? You need to keep your immunity strong. It's that simple. You need to boost the effectiveness of your fabulous infection-fighting white blood cells named intraepithelial lymphocytes which are the first line of defence against incoming pathogens. You need a rainbow diet, making sure you add blueberries as they have been proven to almost double your natural killer cells which are vital members of your immune system's first response team against viruses and cancer cells.

Suicide and Depression

According to the World Health Organization over one million people commit suicide each year. That is about one death every 40 seconds or 3000 per day. For each individual that takes his or her own life, an estimated 20 more attempt to do so. Depression is the leading cause of suicide, and of course if you or anyone you know is experiencing suicidal thoughts, you should seek professional help as soon as possible. But lifestyle choices and the foods that you consume can have a massive impact on how you feel mentally. Adding an abundance of greens to your diet can be helpful due to their high chlorophyll content. Chlorophyll is the green molecule in plant cells that absorb sunlight during photosynthesis. It not only provides the plant with energy, but can boost human energy too. It helps restore the antioxidant content of the blood stream and prevents the digestive system from absorbing toxins, which can help in cases of depression. Often when I have tested clients that are depressed, they have a great deal of toxins in the blood, making them feel awful. Once you use foods to help remove and restore the person's mood it can start to lift.

Saffron, the spice, is found to be amazingly effective at treating depression. It's high in carotenoids and B vitamins that help increase levels of serotonin and other chemicals in the brain that are associated with depression. It is thought that saffron extract is as effective as an anti-depressant medication in treating people with major depression. Curcumin is also thought to help. The pigment that gives turmeric its yellow-orange colour is well known for its powerful antioxidant and anti-inflammatory properties. As there is a connection between inflammation and depression this is a great remedy to reduce symptoms.

There is one thing that I didn't know whether to mention or not, purely because the last thing I want to do is cause any offence or disrespect people in the medical profession. As I said earlier, I have doctor friends and doctors in my family, so I have a great deal of love and gratitude for the profession. However, the reason I have chosen to include this information is because I think we all have the right to be informed, so we can make potentially life-changing decisions as and when we need to. There is a reason why it is so important for us to take care of ourselves, and why I say repeatedly that prevention is far better than cure. According to Dr Michael Greger, getting a routine chest CT scan is estimated to inflict the same cancer risk as smoking 700 cigarettes. Or that maybe one person in every 270 may develop cancer after a single CT angiogram. How about medication for high cholesterol, blood pressure, and blood thinning drugs? Apparently, the chance of even high-risk patients benefiting from them is typically less than 5% over a period of five years. The question is this: are we overestimating the power of pills and procedures to ward off death and disability?

Did you know that the third leading cause of mortality in the US, responsible for more than 225,000 deaths annually, is medical blunders? It's shocking to hear this for the first time, and it gives me absolutely no pleasure to share this information, but due to infections in hospitals, unnecessary surgery, receiving the wrong medication, or adverse side effects from the right medication, the facts and figures are alarming. A very good friend of mine experienced first-hand how things can change in a second. His sister went into hospital for a routine operation on her knee when she was 14 years old. He was 15. His sister never returned home, dying from complications due to the operation. He has never recovered from this traumatic event. These things happen, and I know that all hospitals across the world are working harder than ever to reduce medical errors and contain infections. They are fighting an almost impossible war and the nurses, doctors, and just about everyone else that works in the health establishment are devoted and incredible.

But we must look into the true issues. We are still failing to address the root cause of many diseases. Our hospitals are brilliant at fixing broken bones and curing infections, but what about preventative medicine? Preventing, reversing, stabilizing, detecting warning signs, nutritional changes … these are all things we should be striving towards. That's why we should take control of our own bodies and take full responsibility for our own health, and I hope I can help you to see how you can do this.

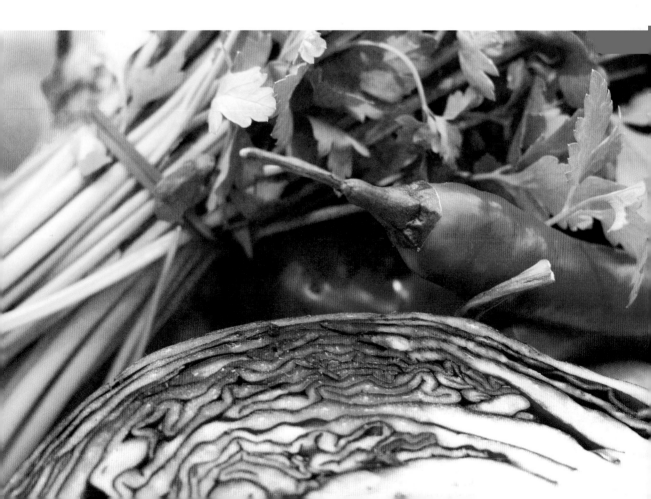

CHAPTER 6

TIME TO CLEAN OUT THE CRAPOLA!

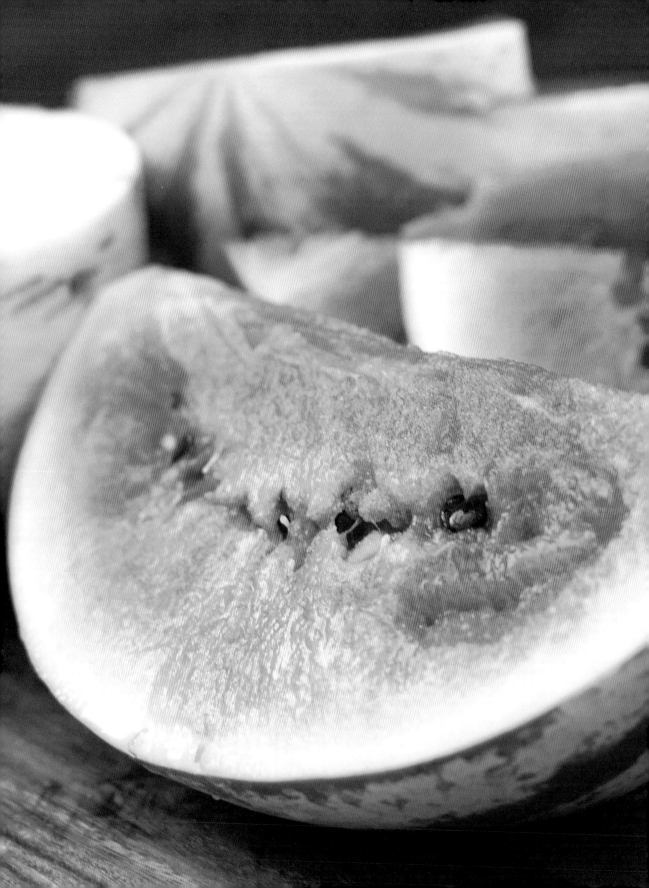

Let me get one thing straight with you all. Dis-ease (meaning the body is not in harmony) in the body of any, any, any, any (I can't emphasize that enough) description is not OK. If you are suffering in some way, and your body is functioning at a low-level vibration because you have stomach ache, a headache, are bloated, foggy in the brain, or some ill-effect is making you feel less than energetic, possibly even making you feel like you are treading the treacle of life instead of gliding over fields of daffodils (OK, a slight exaggeration of a fantasy perfect life) you need to do something about it. I see people day in, day out, that have been suffering for years from migraines or digestive complaints such as irritable bowel, acid reflux, bloating, or excess gas. Or they may be afflicted with constant urinary/bladder infections or erectile dysfunction. Or some sort of breathing issue, such as asthma, allergies, coughs, and chest infections. Or stuffy noses, throat infections, or aching bones and joints. Or chilblains, cold sores, constipation, vomiting, vertigo, varicose veins, tinnitus, thyroid issues, swollen glands. Or skin complaints such as psoriasis, eczema, dryness, irritation, or ovarian cysts, thrush, mouth ulcers, miscarriages, menopausal symptoms, leg cramps, anaemia, haemorrhoids, gout, fibromyalgia, memory loss. The list goes on and on, and I have seen it all.

What I find alarming though is that because so many people are suffering from what I call the 'common complaints', when they realize many others have the same illness, they suddenly think it can't be that bad, and resign themselves to a life of visits to the doctor and pill popping. NO! There is no safety in numbers. You must break free.

My point is this: do not be a sheep. Stick to your guns and do what you believe to be right for you. Break free of the general thinking and take care of your own body. If you give it what it needs it will thank you so much in the end, and give you back your life, your energy, your zest, and your control. Always remember you are the driver of your body! Almost all the ailments I have mentioned can be helped, if not cleared up completely, if you clean up your diet. And I mean really clear up … properly, like a house move where you remove all the crap, dust it out, scrub all the carpets, chuck out and remove the debris, and replace with new and shiny things. You will be very surprised at your new enthusiasm for life.

Here are the rules for your clean-up.

Stop Putting Rubbish Into Your Body and Start Putting the Right Nutrition In

This is a very simplistic thing to say. 'If only it were that easy,' I hear you scream! Well, it doesn't need to be complicated. Slowly, over the coming weeks, if you want to start making changes, you need to start pulling out some of the bad stuff that you eat. It depends on where you are already on the health scale, but if you eat fast food four times per week and drink six pints every night, then I would start by reducing the amounts that you consume. Or if you already have a great diet and want to maintain health or enhance your energy, start by adding a few more superfoods.

Know and Understand the Two Main Reasons Why Disease Manifests

You are nutrient deficient – in other words, you simply do not have enough of the good stuff going in on a daily basis. If you start to view food differently and use it as a tool to help you at every single mealtime, and every single snack, then you will start to shift your mindset, which makes new challenges much easier. Every single thing that you put in your mouth has the potential to make you feel amazing and energized or foggy and sluggish. Take a quick recap on what you have eaten today. Is it good enough for your precious body? Did you really deserve that chocolate bar that added a few more pounds to your butt, challenged your liver just a little bit more, and made you feel sleepy an hour after eating it? Or did you deserve that ripe juicy mango, that is low in calories and high in fibre which will help to keep your beautiful intestines clean. It also contains real folate, vitamins B6, C, and A, so your eyes look whiter, your skin glows, and your body purrs from the antioxidants you have just drenched it in. Do you see the difference in the choices that you made today?

You are too acidic/toxic – ditch the junk! What is so appealing about highly processed foods anyway? If you look at a nice green juicy apple and then a slab of sliced processed ham, in the real world what looks more appealing? Well, the secret to all those foods that we supposedly love, such as crisps, biscuits, cakes, and chocolate is because they are loaded with a trifecta of fat, sodium, and sugar with plenty of extra ingredients that function to preserve and improve their appearance. These foods are carefully engineered to achieve a perfect balance and produce pleasure so you can't help but keep eating them. I have seen many clients who describe their eating habits as out of control and this is the reason why: eating these man-made hyperpalatable foods produces pleasure-providing opioids in the human body.

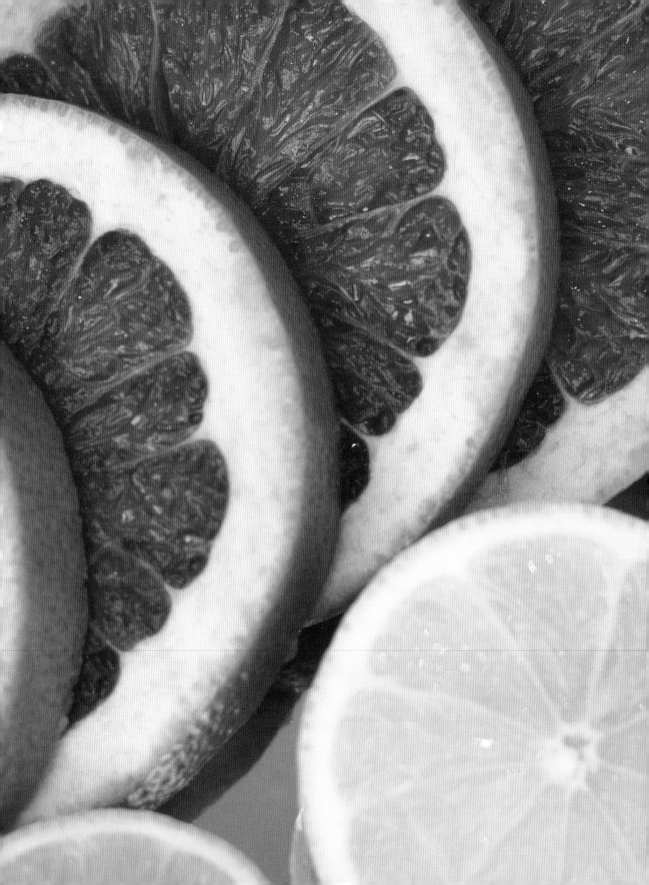

There have been trials carried out on laboratory animals where they actually preferred the intense sweetness from food to cocaine. These animals became quickly addicted to sugar and demonstrated significant withdrawal symptoms, including the shakes and anxious behaviour, when it was removed. Individuals participating in 'comfort eating', or as I like to call it 'junk food eating', are looking for a certain sensation of pleasure or relief not unlike abusers of nicotine, alcohol, or drugs such as heroin or cocaine. When you get into this behaviour the same terms are used about eating – it's called 'using' food rather than 'eating' food. We need to ask ourselves the very important question: how is this allowed in the food industry? How are mass food producers allowed to concoct certain foods which produce similar addictive effects to drugs?

So is food addiction real? Yes, I think it is. I think it's too easy for someone to feel emotional about something and reach for that bag of crisps because they want a lift that very second. Before you know it, you have trawled your way through the entire packet and then your feelings of self-loathing go through the roof! Not only do you feel sick from eating too much salt and fat but that then provokes angry feelings, which sparks yet more toxicity within the body. Other junk foods such as processed meats, sausages, bacon, and salami are all classed as everyday foods. Really? Who made that normal? Then there the doughnuts and cakes that every office purchases for birthday celebrations. What's wrong with bringing a basket of delicious fruits for everyone to feast on? In the olden days, when you got sick, people would bring you grapes and bananas. That's because we instinctively knew it would contribute to making you better. And it did!

Then there are pizzas and chips, and fast food restaurants everywhere. The word 'junk' refers to something that is both extra and useless, and that is exactly what junk food is. Look at what is in front of you. What are you about to eat? Does it have a purpose for your beautiful body, or is it going to back up the crapola so much that you explode. Junk food makes you tired! FACT! It makes you feel full and satisfied temporarily, and then you want more, because it hasn't actually satisfied you for very long, and that's because of the lack of nutrients. When the body is nutrient rich you shouldn't crave anything, because you have all that you need. Junk food lacks nutrients and causes havoc in your body and if you eat it on a daily basis it will affect your everyday performance levels.

Teenagers in particular have a great deal of hormonal changes going on in their bodies, which makes them susceptible to mood swings and behavioural issues. These are two reasons we have an epidemic of depressed teenagers: because of the lack of physical movement and the increase in eating junk food daily. It actually puts their risk of depression up by over 50%. It's so simple though. They are basically not getting enough of the good stuff and clearly getting too much of the bad stuff. Would you ever run your Rolls Royce on nitroglycerin? No, because it would blow up. So why eat junk? It makes no sense. You are simply filling your body up with muck as there is a serious lack of fibre making it difficult for the digestive system. Then people can suffer from reflux or irritable bowel syndrome.

Just imagine this … because junk food is deep fried all the oil gets sloshed around and stuck, causing irritation of the stomach lining and inflammation of the intestines and bowel. The reason you want more of it is because it is high in refined sugars putting your metabolism under great stress. It causes your pancreas to secrete more insulin in order to prevent a dramatic spike in your blood sugar levels, causing irritation and more cravings when you have a blood sugar crash! This then affects brain function, behaviour, and immunity in as little as a week of eating the stuff. Not only that … because of the high fat and sugar content it massively increases your risk of heart disease, cancer, kidney disease, and liver damage. Colorectal cancer is related to consuming processed food.

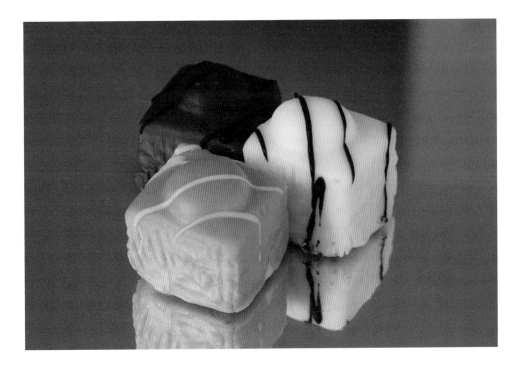

Cut Out the Coffee and Stimulants

If you have health challenges and want to be as clean as you can be in order to achieve great health then you need to consider the following. There are lots of studies to report that caffeine is good for you. Well, you can make up your own mind, but my point of view is this. If you experience withdrawal symptoms when you do not have something in your diet for one day, you are addicted. Plain and simple. The reason you get a head-ache when you give up caffeine, whether that be your energy drink, coffee, or tea, is because of the sudden increased circulation to the brain when blood flow is no longer constricted. When you consume your cup of caffeine there is a widespread constriction of vital organ blood vessels, which actually decreases circulation and oxygen supply by up to 30%. As a stimulant it will increase your heart rate, raise your blood pressure, and form an acidic environment for all your healthy cells to bathe in. This is far from ideal, as your cells need an alkaline fluid to thrive. Alkaline and health-enhancing foods are best to keep our bodies happy and maintain an anti-inflammatory environment. Don't be fooled either into thinking that decaf coffee is a better choice as this causes even more acidity and most of us, to be real, are acidic enough. Too much caffeine has been linked to calcium loss, contributing to osteoporosis and bone issues. Roasted coffee beans have also been linked to cancer because they form a potent carcinogen called benzoprene when roasted, which is said to increase the risk of pancreatic cancer.

Energy drinks stress our bodies out by overworking the adrenal glands, and the stress hor-mones can remain in the body for up to 18 hours, which promotes the production of cortisol. Too much cortisol reduces our immune function and decreases the energy that we need for the healthy repair and renewal of our 100 trillion cells. When you try to remove energy sub-stances, not only can it give you a headache, you can feel fatigued, irritable, discontented, depressed, and even have flu-like symptoms such as nausea and vomiting. The effects of withdrawal can be so powerful that as soon as you reintroduce the substance, all your horrid symptoms disappear, which is why so many people cannot live without these substances.

So what are the good points? Are there antioxidants in coffee? Or in chocolate? Yes, of course, but they also exist in cocaine and heroin too. Forget the energy caffeine drinks altogether. They contain so many other toxic ingredients that I would eliminate them. The polyphenols found in coffee that provide you with your antioxidants are found in so many other plant-based foods too. Vegetables such as bok choy and mustard greens, and the skin of grapes have it in full supply. The difference is that whole foods can provide you with the very same thing, but also with fibre and high amounts of quality vitamins, minerals, and essential fatty acids, therefore giving you the balance that you need for good health. Do not compromise your health, instead nourish your body.

Eliminate Dairy from Your Diet

I have friends that are farmers, and I don't like broaching this subject because people's livelihoods are at stake. However, I have to be honest and speak as I find. In my clinics I can only say that there are numerous disease processes I have witnessed that have been massively helped by cutting dairy out of the diet. A person can feel almost immediate relief, especially when it comes to inflammation, congestion, or pain. The question I get asked all the time is 'where do I get my calcium from?' Let's set the record straight, because we are so preconditioned to think we need this drink in order to keep us strong. Most of the calcium present in cow's milk is useless to the body. In order for calcium to be absorbed, magnesium must be present in equal quantities. Remember I said that's why vitamins and minerals are much better consumed as nature intended because we have all that we need to absorb the goodness. One cup of milk contains 291 milligrams of calcium and 33 milligrams of magnesium, so only about 11% of the calcium can be absorbed. Milk contains a high level of protein, and, like meat and caffeine, is extremely acid forming. Then the body must have the resources to neutralize this. Most of us don't have enough alkaline minerals to do the job, so what happens? The body leaches from the bones in order to get the alkaline substances that it needs. In other words, it robs minerals from your bones when you do not provide it with enough, due to your dietary choices. This results in bones dissolving in order to release the necessary minerals to neutralize the acids. So milk not only offers very little in protecting against osteoporosis, it may very well contribute to the disease that we are trying to prevent!

The highest rate of hip fractures worldwide occur among the populations that consume … you've guessed it … the most dairy! The USA consumes more milk than anywhere else in the world and has the highest incidence of osteoporosis. The lowest rates are found amongst people who eat little or no dairy. And think about it.

Where do the cows get their calcium from anyway? From the green grass that they eat!

Greens are one of the richest sources of chlorophyll in the world, and as magnesium is the central atom of the chlorophyll molecule it makes greens the richest sources of minerals needed for calcium absorption. So, what do you think you should be consuming in order to prevent osteoporosis? Greens, greens, and more greens such as broccoli, kale, spinach, and collard! In abundance. Cow's milk, including organic milk, contains more than 50 active hormones, a ton of allergens, and loads of fat and cholesterol. It's said the recommended three glasses per day contain the same amount of cholesterol as in 53 slices of bacon! Other ingredients your white stuff could include are antibiotics, blood, pus, faeces, bacteria, viruses, pesticides, and herbicides. Needless to say, milk has been at the forefront of many studies relating breast, ovarian, prostate, and colon cancers to its intake, as well as MS and diabetes. Don't even go there with raw milk either. It is promoted as having enzymes needed to digest the milk, but in reality, it contains dangerous bacteria such as salmonella and listeria to name only a few.

Basically, nature did not intend for us to drink milk after weaning, especially not that of another species, and it can contribute to serious disease. Officially dairy is right up there, being linked to serious diseases. Think about this … is it a normal process to suck milk from another species? Just because it's the farmer milking the cow, doesn't make it any better than you taking a chair over and putting your head right under the cow's belly and having a good old suck. Sounds gross, right? Well, it is, if you think about it logically. And when I say dairy, I mean all dairy. Milk, cream, cheese, cottage cheese, Greek yoghurt, kefir. You name it. When you consume such foods, they produce more mucus in your body, therefore creating gloopier blood. Gloopier blood presents health challenges like clogging of the arteries, potentially leading to premature death.

Reduce or Ditch the Meat

The fact is that people are getting sicker, younger. We live in a very polluted world and one of the most essential things to stay healthy and energetic is to try and keep the body from being toxic. When we eat meat, we are carrying more heavy metals, more antibiotics, more harmful hormone-related chemicals and toxins right back into the body, and if it takes something like three days to leave the body those toxins are just going to accumulate. Our bodies were not designed to eat meat. And for those of you that think chicken, turkey, and duck are a safe bet, think again. These meats contain more saturated fat, linking them to heart disease and strokes, and have been linked to breast cancer in some studies. This is not to say it is the only cause of breast cancer but it is being found to be a major contributor. Most meats are injected with various steroids and female hormones to fatten them up as the fatter the animal the more money you can get for your meat. But when you eat the meat you, too, are ingesting the hormones, creating all sorts of carnage in your body. In higher meat-eating communities it has been suggested that there are more murders, more rapes, and more incest, and this can surely be linked to higher oestrogen and testosterone being pumped into your body.

But meat is the only way for you to get protein, right? Wrong! 100 calories of steak provides you with 5.4 grams of protein. How would you feel if I were to tell you that

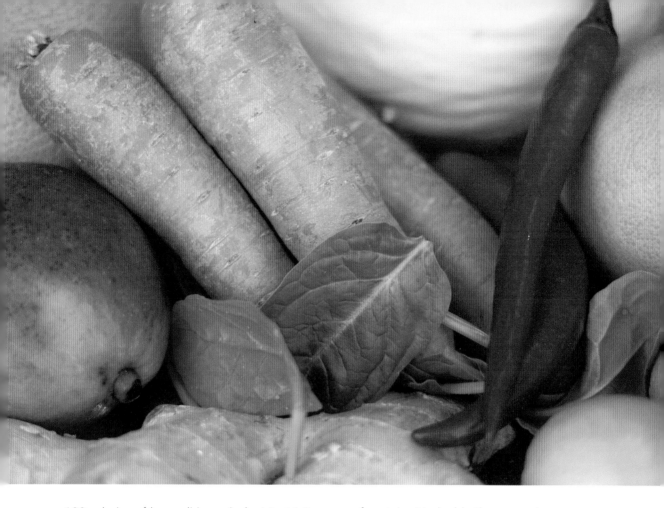

100 calories of broccoli is equivalent to 11.2 grams of protein. It's double the amount in steak! Crazy, hey! So why are we led to believe that we need meat? The meat industry is big business. Think about cows as an example. They get big and strong by eating grass. That is where they get their protein from, so why can't you get yours from greens? Half a million people every year will have their chests opened up and a vein taken from their leg and sewn into their coronary artery because it's blocked. Change your lifestyle choices and maybe you wouldn't need to have this extreme and life-threatening surgery. Meat of all descriptions is acidic to the body, and a body living in an acidic environment is at higher risk of disease. Meat causes inflammation, raises insulin growth factors, and causes insulin resistance, leading to diabetes, and disrupts the endocrine pathways, which is linked to cancers and obesity.

Not only is it potentially harming you to consume too much meat, but it could be the biggest cause of global warming too. If you want to help your planet and care about global warming, then it might be good to cut down or cut out altogether your consumption of meat. The global livestock industry produces more greenhouse gas emissions than cars, planes, trains, and ships combined. Our attention has been very much on deforestation over the years, and rightly so, but preventing catastrophic warming is dependent on tackling our worldwide meat and dairy consumption, too. Eating a plant-based diet is probably the best way you can reduce your impact on Planet Earth, not just for greenhouse gases, but also global acidification, plus land and water use. Life is all about choices and information.

Ditch the Fish

It's hard to comprehend, but the entire planet is contaminated. The ocean contains a plethora of pollutants and toxins such as mercury, plastics, pharmaceutical drugs, and a complex amount of other highly health-challenging chemicals. You take the drugs, pee in the toilet, flush the toilet, which then takes that water into the rivers, lakes, and streams, where it gets dumped into the sea. Man-made pharmaceutical drugs can take thousands of years to break down, and Prozac (one of the most common antidepressants) is said to be creating havoc amongst dolphins, sharks, whales, and fish. Because of toxicity in their bodies, they have been reported to be beaching themselves in confusion instead of swimming into the ocean. Fish hold onto the toxins found in the water and then we eat them. We must ask ourselves if this is a good choice if we want great health? While they do have health-enhancing properties such as being rich in omega 3, it is becoming more and more debatable how effective this is because of the amount of pollutants they are carrying.

Reduce the Alcohol or Stop Completely

OK, OK, I know I do like a few bubbles every now and again, but I am known amongst my party gals as the 'lightweight'! In all seriousness I have very strong views on the UK's drinking culture. In fact … I *hate* it! I am sorry for all you die-hard UK fans. I really love my country and am proud to be British on so many levels, but when it comes to drinking, and I am having a discussion with any other nationality, I want to run as far away from admitting that I'm British as is humanly possible. I have been in proper hardcore drinking countries such as Russia and Lithuania on corporate training events, and boy, they can drink. But they start to tell me stories of how they cannot keep up with us Brits when it comes to all-night sessions. What? This is not something to be proud of.

When I was growing up, I remember being desperate to be able to tolerate drink a little better, so I could stay at the bar with my friends, shot for shot. Little did I know at the time that being the tiniest out of all my friends (5ft 2in, and that's pushing it!) I literally didn't have the body build to be able to tolerate large volumes of alcohol in this way, so it wasn't my fault that I passed out quicker than everyone else. It was human biology! The human body is made up of more water than anything else. The water is mostly stored in the blood so the taller and heavier a person is, the bigger their circulation, and the more water they carry. When alcohol enters the bloodstream, it gets diluted by water, lessening its impact. Then, the more water there is, the more alcohol gets diluted. So, it's official, the larger your body is, the more watered down your drinks become. This can also explain why men are generally better at holding their booze than us ladies. A man is 60% water, and a woman 55%, so even with equal body mass it would be an uneven contest! Sorry ladies, but as much as you may want to argue this point, we are just not as well equipped to tolerate alcohol in the way a man's body is. And we are also prone to more liver toxicity and other complications from drinking to excess.

Generally, though, drinking lots of alcohol is just not great for us. We all know that next-day feeling. The headache, feeling tired and groggy, not to mention the detrimental effect on our appearance. It also increases our risk of other, much more serious diseases including breast cancer, oral cancers, heart disease, strokes, and cirrhosis of the liver. It has a detrimental effect on our mental health, can lead to depression, affect fertility, and shrink our brain. There are conflicting studies to suggest that a glass of alcohol used as a relaxant can have benefits, but the risk of increasing serious disease is so apparent now that you have to ask yourself, is it worth it? So if you like a few glasses every now and then you are not going to get shot down in flames. Just make sure you are balancing it with a lorryload of alkalizing fruits and vegetables the next day to put the body back in order. However, if you are regularly binge drinking or drinking several glasses every day, you need to seriously reconsider your lifestyle choices, and the reasons behind your drinking may also need to be addressed.

Smoking

There are so few people that actually still do but if you participate in the odd puff here's what it does to you. Nicotine is an addictive substance, I think we all know that by now. It stimulates dopamine in the brain, which is responsible for pleasurable sensations such as boosting your mood, alleviating minor depression, and giving you an overall sense of well-being. But, the more you smoke, the more your nerve cells become immune to the pleasure, so as with any drug, you need more and more to get that high. While smoking may make you feel good temporarily, it's slowly killing your body. It is the leading preventable cause of death in the world. Let's start with the bad breath first, and the yellow stains on your teeth. No one wants that now, do they? It also leads to premature wrinkles, gum disease, and tooth loss. So what's the attraction? Plus, your poor immunity gets a hammering every time you have a little puff.

People who smoke from a young age are more likely to continue smoking into adulthood, which could eventually lead to heart issues and increase their risk of stroke and permanent respiratory issues, in turn leading to progressive loss of function and a condition known as emphysema. This disease causes the air sacs in your lungs to deteriorate, reducing the surface area which makes it hard to breathe. I think all children should be taken to hospitals where you can see people living with emphysema. My great aunt, whom I really loved, had this condition and it was horrific to watch someone deteriorate in this way. Almost suffocating to death. And please don't be fooled into vaping either. Although e-cigarettes do not produce smoke, the vapour is not harmless. The aerosol from the e-cigarettes contains many potentially harmful chemicals, including lead and other heavy metals. It also has flavourings including diacetyl which has been linked to lung disease. There have not been nearly enough studies on these devices yet, but I can only say one thing. The *only* substance we are meant to breathe into our lungs is fresh air! Full stop! That's it. Nothing else is safe enough for you to dabble with.

Remove the White Stuff

Sugar is considered by some to be as bad as heroin in the way it is processed and used, sugar dulls the brain, impairs organ function, strips the body of calcium, taps mineral reserves, contributes to obesity, depression, and cellular death. It is officially a poison. Refined sugar is stripped of all its nutrients, and then we are back to the same scenario as the milk. In order for our body to process this substance that has no nutrients, it must rob its own reserves of vital vitamins and minerals. It will target calcium in the bones and teeth because calcium is the primary mineral the body uses to neutralize high acid levels in the cells. Then there is a danger of being left with toxic minerals when there is not enough calcium left to fight the acid. That may lead in turn to dental plaque, osteoporosis, arthritis, kidney stones, and hardening of the arteries.

You see sugar alters our blood chemistry, and critical enzymes are unable to do their job when minerals are depleted. When this imbalance is created our digestion is all over the place and our immune system weakens. Sugar is very difficult for the body to break down, even as little as a tablespoon creates a strain on the body and it takes a lot of effort from magnesium, sodium, and potassium to restore the balance. With a daily diet of refined sugar, now in fatty acid form, the liver begins to swell, causing a backup. So it has to go into the blood which then stores it in inactive places such as your butt, belly, thighs, and stomach. Sugar kills off the good bacteria and causes deficiencies in B vitamins (the energy-enhancing vitamins) which can disturb sleep, increase memory fog, and in the long term can lead to depression and dementia.

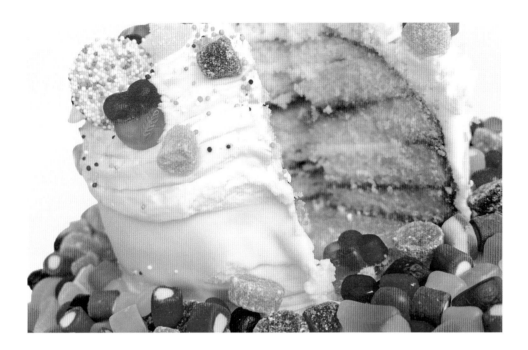

Take our average breakfast for an example of how much sugar we take in at one sitting. Sometimes half the ingredients in cereal are made of sugar and 2/3 of a cup of fruit-flavoured yoghurt can be loaded with up to 2 teaspoons of sugar. A bottle of orange juice can contain 10 teaspoonsful. And that's meant to be the healthy option! The rule is to avoid anything with refined sugar. Have a gorgeous health-enhancing green juice for your breakfast instead. You will feel energized, invigorated, and focused for the day. You certainly don't need a mix of processed junk to send you into a fog before your day has even started. And please don't go for the same foods, but just the sugar-free version. Many artificial sweeteners have been potentially linked to all sorts of serious diseases, including cancer, and if they were so good anyway, why isn't everyone super skinny? If you make sure you feed your body with excellent nourishment, your sugar cravings will naturally reduce anyway. It's a work in progress, and something that is hard to do because of the constant temptation that surrounds us, but it is possible to kick this habit for good.

Remove Stress – Get It Out of Your Life!

For those of you in your twenties, I don't think you will understand what I mean by this. I don't mean that in an offensive or patronizing manner, but when you are twenty you are just loving life and living it to the max with millions of friends, parties, and socializing. This is the way it's meant to be for the majority of us! I know I am generalizing here, and not everyone is the same, but basically that was me and most of my friends in our twenties and it was fabulous. I would let any old Tom, Dick, or Harry into my life. Energy vampires, happy laughter givers, bitches from hell, adorable kind souls, loud offensive nutters, quiet and shy introverts, and vivacious extroverts. They were all there. As many different types of people as possible! Bring them on! Then, in your thirties, you wise up a little to the people you love and start to value people more and realize what they bring to you and you to them. You might pop out a few little bambinos or not as the case may be, you might adopt, get IVF, buy five dogs, a houseboat, and a 4x4, but by the time you reach your forties you are beginning to question things and people more than before. Material things begin to have less meaning.

I am not quite so brave yet, but my friends that are in their fifties are harsh! Basically, watch out world … They are spitting out friends, husbands, wives, girlfriends, boy-friends, toy boys, puppies without a care in the world. They take no prisoners! They have learnt that finally they need no crap in their lives. If someone has a negative effect on you, ditch them. They don't care who it is but know that you no longer have to 'people please' because it causes you stress. Negative people bring negative situations, and negative situations cause disharmony to your precious beautiful bodies. Stress will cause you harm and manifest your disease process, affecting your gut, skin (could be the major cause of eczema and psoriasis), hair, nails, heart and lungs, mind and sanity. It affects your muscles and joints, your ability to think rationally and make decisions correctly, and causes a high level of anxiety and sleepless nights. It can affect your sex life, make you feel depressed, and crush your confidence. Make a list of all the things that are stressing you out and remove them from your life. No mercy and no prisoners. And if you can't fix it or get rid of it, it's not worth worrying about. As the Dalai Lama said: 'If a problem is fixable, if a situation is such that you can do something about it, then there is no need to worry. If it's not fixable, then there is no help in worrying. There is no benefit in worrying whatsoever.'

Get Moving

I have spent a lot of time in the library for peace and quiet whilst writing. At my regular haunt, there is a beautiful sweeping staircase leading up to the quiet area on the first floor and I cannot tell you how many people I have seen use the lift to get up to this floor. It's one thing if you have a medical condition, disability, or injury and you can't climb the stairs, but if not, get your lazy little bootie walking up those stairs. The impor-tance of exercise is obvious and we have covered that in Chapter 4. But make decisions every day that are going to get you moving just that little bit more. Vacuum your house frequently, mow the lawn, take an extra flight of stairs just for the sake of it. Park your car further away from the ticket machine, park two extra blocks away from your work, walk to get your groceries instead of getting the tube or the subway.

When my beautiful daughter and I were in New York City recently, we walked everywhere. You can see so much more and get your bearings better in any city, and I guarantee you that everything's a lot closer than you think. We just get conditioned into habits that are difficult to break. Make time to walk to work. Factor that into your day and keep your trainers in your bag at all times so there are no excuses. It's a fact that sedentary lifestyles increase all causes of mortality, double the risk of cardiovascular disease, obesity, and diabetes, and increase your risk of high blood pressure, colon and numerous other types of cancers, and your risk of depression and anxiety. It's plain and simple … get moving as much as you can.

Ditch the Medication

I'm getting into dangerous territory here, and I know I must be careful what I say. Some people have to be on medication for specific health issues, but all medication without exception is challenging to your liver and will result to some level of toxicity within your body. If you are taking numerous medications, prescription or otherwise, once you reach five or more different types you are entering into something called polypharmacy and the risk of harmful effects, drug interactions, and hospitalization begins to increase. The craziest thing of all is that the people that are the sickest take the most drugs, but they are the most vulnerable to unpredictable effects, not only on the disease and their well-being but also interactions between the drugs themselves. Then the more you take, the more drugs you need to counteract the side effects of the drugs you are already taking. Madness!

As we get older the brain becomes more sensitive to drug effects, and medications stay longer in the body due to the fact that we have less muscle and more body fat. Our bodies contain less water so medications can become more concentrated, and our liver and kidneys do not process medications as effectively as they did when we were younger. Regardless of your age or your disease, check that you really do need to be taking the medication that you on, or as many pills as you are taking. Question your doctor if you are not sure why you are taking it, and make sure it is necessary for you and your disease. Gone are the days where you said 'yes sir, no sir'. Doctors don't know everything, and nor do I, but it is your right to question and make the best decisions that you can for your own body. Take control, get all the facts, and make sure you are not polluting your environment (body) any more than you have to.

Don't Avoid the Sun

We have been told for so long to avoid the sun because it's bad for us, and yes, the harsh UV rays are dangerous if you are baking yourself for hours on end laying in the midday sun. But a burst of sunshine with no sunscreen on is a breath of fresh air to your body – literally! Sunshine boosts your levels of serotonin, the body's natural happy hormone. Just 5 to 10 minutes of exercise outdoors (a walk in the park will do) is enough to make you feel less stressed and happier. Not only that, serotonin can act as a natural appetite suppressant helping you to maintain a healthy weight. High levels of vitamin D can boost your memory and protect you against cancer, help to increase your fertility and maintain strong bones and gorgeous skin. Being woken up gradually by the sun's natural light switches off melatonin, the hormone that stimulates sleep, which improves your energy and mood for the day, so get rid of the blackout blinds and let the natural light wake you.

People who do not get enough sunlight have altered cellular defence mechanisms that can predispose them to excessive inflammation, which can result in autoimmune diseases such as asthma, psoriasis, dermatitis, multiple sclerosis, lupus, type 1 diabetes, and inflammatory bowel disease. Basically, do not avoid the sun completely. Your body needs it. A little sunlight every day (even if you live in a cold dark country you can still get vitamin D on a cloudy day) can reduce the number of activated cells that lead to inflammation and doing so you help reduce your risk of serious diseases.

Do not Compromise on Sleep

I am a bit of a night owl, and always have been. I do my best writing when everyone else in my household is in bed. I guess there is an element of comfort knowing that everyone is safe under one roof and when I know my children are safe and happy all is OK with my world. But I also love early morning runs, and I know I need eight hours' sleep in order to function at my best, so getting this balance is a challenge for me. Some people genuinely need less than the average eight hours, but any less than six and you are getting into deprivation territory. However, if I go to bed at 1 or 2 a.m. I do not feel that great the next day, even if I do get the same number of hours. Why is this? The sleep you get before midnight has been scientifically proven to be better for you as it can restore your body more efficiently. Every hour of sleep you get before midnight is worth three times as much and better for your overall health than the after-midnight sleep. Before electricity everyone went to bed early and woke up early. That's because the sun helps guide your sleep/wake cycle, making your daily life much easier to manage.

While you sleep your immune system releases a type of small protein called cytokines. If you are sick or injured these cytokines help fight body trauma, infection, and inflammation. That's why our immune system becomes compromised if we don't get enough sleep. Sometimes you can go to bed with a headache and wake up without it! It's a small miracle! Your stress hormone cortisol also decreases while you sleep which gives your body the welcome rest that it needs in order to set about all its restoring and repairing of your luscious little cells. When you are deprived of sleep, your sympathetic nervous system activity increases, which is also mirrored by an increase in blood pressure. Investigations are still going on to see if there is a relationship between decreased sleep duration and the increased risk of heart disease, which I think is very likely. There are numerous hormones released while you are sleeping, such as melatonin, which is secreted by the pineal gland, an important process that helps to control your sleep patterns.

People that do shift work can get really messed-up sleep cycles and this can take a negative toll on their health. Around 10% of shift workers have a diagnosed 'shift work sleep disorder' which involves ill effects from sleep deprivation. They can experience fatigue, weight gain, lack of concentration, high cholesterol, and memory issues. In fact, anyone who doesn't get enough sleep can suffer damaging effects over time. Being more

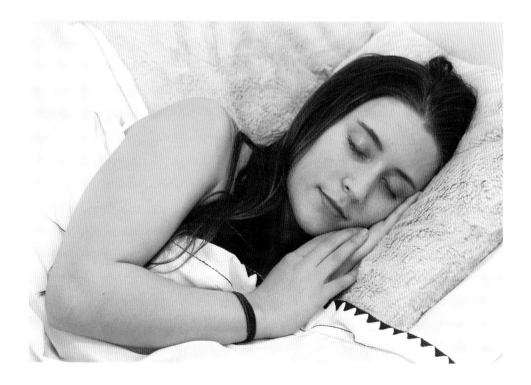

emotional, moody, or angry is a classic symptom of sleep deprivation. Your body becomes less resilient against viruses and infections and releases more insulin, increasing the risk of diabetes. Your chances of having an accident are much higher too, making sleep deprivation extremely dangerous in some circumstances. The effects on the brain from lack of sleep are similar to the effects of drinking too much alcohol. Yet drowsy driving does not get nearly as much attention as drunk driving. Drivers who sleep less than four hours the night before have 11 times the crash rates of drivers who slept seven or more hours a night.

I remember coming back from Australia a few years ago. I had never really suffered from jet lag to that extent before, but it was utterly horrendous. I had to do a simple one-hour journey to work two days after returning home from our trip, and it wasn't until I got in the car that I realized how disorientated I felt. I had to concentrate on every tiny move I was making. Normally driving a car is an automatic procedure. It was the strangest out-of-body experience I have ever had. Needless to say I got 10 minutes up the road, pulled over, and slowly made my way back home to bed. I felt completely out of control, my coordination was all over the place and my brain was without doubt dangerously out of sync with my body!

And have you ever looked closely in the mirror after a few nights of poor sleep. It ain't pretty! The boost in the human growth hormone from restful sleep is related to an increase in the production of collagen, the protein that gives skin its elasticity and firmness and helps keeps wrinkles at bay. If the only reason you want to get a good night's sleep is because you want to keep your glowing youthful appearance, that's good enough for me. Just know that getting enough sleep is vital for great lasting health and vitality.

Ditch the Microwave

I wish I could leave it there without any explanation, as in my eyes it's utterly unnecessary and not one of us really needs this device in our house. We have enough radiation and pollution bombarding our fabulous bodies at the best of times. Why would you want to cook your food (because it would be convenience food anyway, packaged and processed) in a microwave oven? Yes, I know it's quick, but I believe it zaps the nutrition out of your food like a leach sucking blood. It becomes dead food. And in addition, the non-ionizing radiation of the microwave can cause changes in your blood and heart rate. It's a toxic risk you can do without, despite how safe it is claimed to be. And what exactly do you need it for anyway? To cook your jacket potatoes? To heat up your milk? Organize your meal planning better and cook them in the oven, or heat it on the stove.

Ditch the Mobile Phone at Bedtime

The Californian Department of Public Health, along with many other public health officials, warns that the radio frequency energy emitted from your phone while you sleep could increase your risk of brain cancer and tumours of the acoustic nerve and salivary glands. And in any case, it can interfere with sleep leading to nightmares and regular wakening. If you carry your phone around during the day in your bra or you pop it in your pocket you could be causing far more harm than you realize. Sperm cells can be damaged, and prolonged exposure to mobile phone radiation has been linked to many types of cancers including breast and testicular. The World Health Organization has classified mobile phones and any wireless device as a 2B risk which means they are 'possibly carcinogenic to humans'. Human blood exposure to cell phone radiation has a 300% increase in genetic damage in the form of micronuclei (the name given to the small nuclei that form during cell division). This poses a health threat much greater than that of smoking or asbestos exposure. Anyone that has used a mobile phone continuously for 10 years or more is at a far greater risk of eye and brain cancer, on the side of the head most likely to have had the phone closest too. Switch to aeroplane mode at night, or better still remove your device from your room completely and sleep phone free!

Toxic Cleaning Products Need to Go

Chemicals from many household cleaning products could be harmful to your health, especially your lovely lungs. Asthma and other allergies can be directly worsened by using cleaning chemicals, not to mention the risk of cancer, reproductive disorders, hormone disruption, and neurotoxicity. If something says quite clearly on the label, 'Hazardous to humans', it's not something we should be spraying in the air we breathe on a daily basis. There are a whole range of non-toxic products on the market now, but you can also make your own from extremely simple ingredients. Vinegar, baking soda, and essential oils are all amazing when it comes to a sparkling house. Why put yourself in unnecessary danger when you don't have to? I don't know about you, but if I go into a house or a building where they use plug-in air fresheners, it makes me feel like I can't breathe properly. Using aromatherapy oils to make the place smell wonderful is so much better for your health and can offer therapeutic healing effects too. With a little time, effort, and thought you can easily have non-toxic household products. It's such a simple thing to change, with massive benefits to your health.

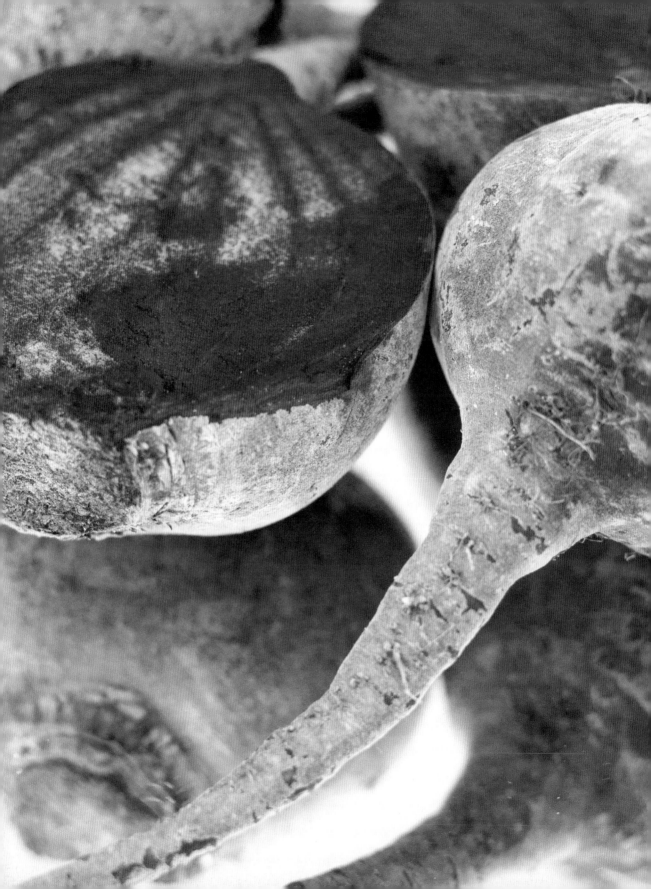

CHAPTER 7

HARDCORE HEALTH FACTS

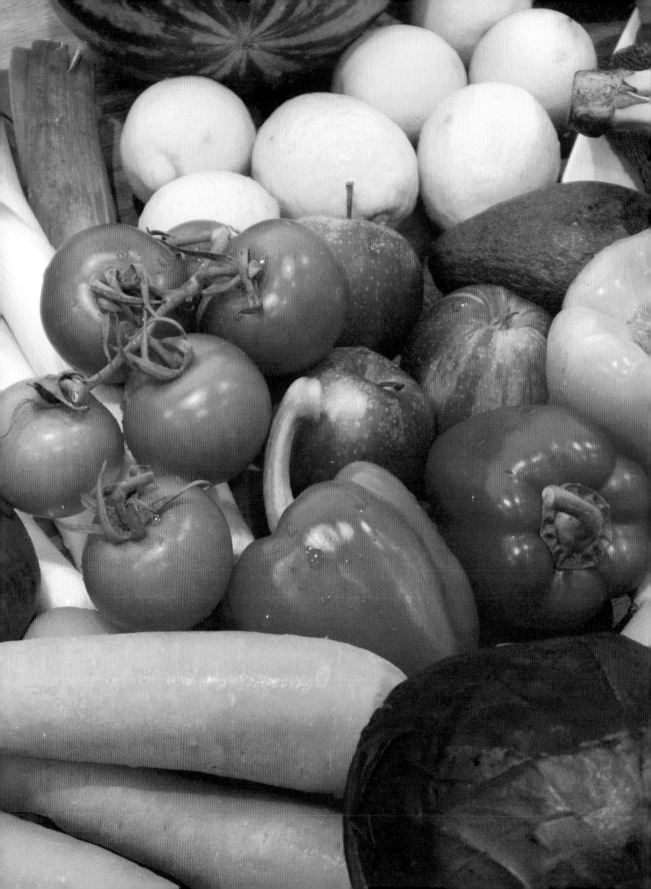

Sometimes it's hard to know how far to take things with food and health, and I do not like to base anything on fear. However, there are some interesting facts that I thought I should share, and I am going to start with this: life is about the survival of the fittest. If you are the undernourished person, or the person that does not exercise enough, if at all, or the person that is miserable in your life and in your work, hates your relationship, and has been through traumas in life, and you decide not to do anything at all about changing your life, your diet, your health-enhancing habits, your mindset and your surroundings … then you are more likely to die of premature ageing and disease; if not, let's face it, you are going to be quite a grump! If you like being miserable, fine, it's your life, but I would encourage you to think again!

Any day, at any time, you can make the right choices. The perfect way to get life force, energy, and feelings of well-being into your precious body is to choose the foods with the most protein, the greatest amounts of vitamins and minerals, the highest source of essential fats, and the best, most natural hormone balancers and providers. Plus the foods with the most phytochemicals and enzymes, and foods which provide you with the optimum amount of oxygen. Nutrition is a relatively new science, believe it or not, and I know that we are all still finding our way. As far as I am aware, the first nutrient was actually discovered right here in my home country, in London, by a man called William Fletcher. He was born in 1872 and was the first scientist to determine that if special factors were removed from foods, disease occurred. He cured beriberi with the use of B vitamins.

Longevity depends on many factors: what you eat, how you think, how you move, what your relationships are like and how much you love your work, or what you do every day to provide your happiness. Overeating is one of the biggest causes of premature death. The people that live the longest, that have the best lives way into old age, are those that do not eat too much and live in a cultural environment that reinforces healthy lifestyles and habits such as a healthy diet and exercise. People living in such settings maintain healthy social relationships, which creates psychological well-being. Seniors are valued and treasured members of society and looked after by the community and their families. I think this is something we get very wrong here in the Western world. Our parents do a wonderful job of nurturing us, sacrificing things and often struggling to pay for food, school fees, etc. and then off we go into the big wide world, earn our money, embark on our careers, and then are too busy or live so far away so we never see them. Then they get old and sick and we stick them in a nursing home. What is that all about?

There have been numerous TV shows and documentaries showing how important it is to have interaction with young children and animals that provide good mental stimulation as well as unconditional love when you reach old age. Loneliness is a killer. Why can't an 80-year-old grandmother be best friends with a 15-year-old boy? They might share the same sense of humour or have similar interests. Why is it that this seems so unlikely? The wisdom that the older generation can give us is priceless. To cast older people off as if they do not matter is nothing but a tragedy. Yes, I know some old people can be grumpy and short-tempered. But what has led them to become that way? Isolation? Loss of a loved one? Every single human being on this planet has a need and a desire to be loved, needed, and wanted, and if you don't have that in your life you are going to deteriorate quite quickly.

I had a very special relationship with my grandparents, and always felt that they were a massive part of my upbringing and the influence on my life. I have tried to maintain that relationship between my own children and my parents as it can offer so much joy and teaching. My father is such a gifted man with many talents, one being his creative hands that can carve anything out of wood. My son would never have been exposed to such learning if he didn't have a great relationship with his grandfather. It's an art that is dying, and one which I treasure, and so does he. My mother is the kindest 'home bird' you will ever meet. Happiest when we are all under her roof eating and talking. She taught my daughter how to bake and how to knit. These are classic skills, but ones which their grandchildren will never forget. For me, having such a good relationship with my grandparents always meant having someone else to confide in, or be answerable to. I was quite a rogue teenager and caused my parents worry for many years. Sometimes my grandparents were easier to talk to about what was going on. Just because there was a 60-year age gap between them and me didn't mean they couldn't understand what was going on. They were so cool and accepting of me, and that made me feel safe and loved, as well as always having my parents' support too, which gave me double the confidence, and double the love! How lucky was I? Appreciating and valuing these precious times is so important.

So if you are old in years but don't want to get mentally old, interact with the young, take yourself off to India, go trekking in the mountains, surround yourself with stimulation and love, or go and live on a cruise ship where you have different people to interact with all day long. Surely it has got to be better than being stuck in one room looking at four walls all day long? We were not meant to live in isolation and, if you do, the chances are your health will deteriorate. The other factor in those places where people live the longest was that they tended to their own communal gardens. Not only did this provide them with organic fresh foods, it also gave them the gift of naturally exercising. They were outside, had to lift, chop, stand up, kneel down, use their arm and legs, and just move around daily. When you tend to a garden you are also giving it love and nurturing, which lifts the human spirit.

Okinawa, in Japan, has the highest life expectancy in the world. They suggest that everyone eats only until they are 80% full instead of gorging themselves. Sardinia in Italy is another place reported to have one of the best life expectancies. They are mostly farmers and shepherds, who have the opportunity to live life in the warmth, walk a lot, take time for leisure, and maintain a positive attitude and sense of humour about life.

Another place ranked right up there for longevity is Loma Linda in California. They focus on healthful habits such as vegetarianism, and, being a religious group, warn heavily against alcohol and smoking. They nurture emotional and spiritual health, prize volunteering, and value their family relationships. They drink plenty of water, eat lots of nuts, and maintain a healthy weight.

It is said that in Nicoya, Costa Rica, a man aged 60 has twice the chance of reaching 90 compared with a man living in the US. Interestingly, they have the lowest rates of cancer and advocate finding their sense of purpose and concentrating on physical activity. They spend lots of time outdoors, sleep eight hours a night, and eat beans, corn, and rice as their staples, as well as drinking water that is naturally high in calcium and magnesium. They also concentrate on family and spiritual time.

Take Greece as another example. Ikaria is a Greek island 35 miles off the coast of Turkey. There is virtually no dementia, half the rate of cardiovascular disease, and at least 20% less cancer. There are famous mineral hot springs, so this place has been a health destination for centuries. Coupled with the Mediterranean diet, they eat lots of wild greens and drink nutritious herbal teas. They take regular naps, and socialize daily, staying active through walking, farming, and fishing. Do you see the pattern that is emerging here? These are all habits that we need to learn from and make efforts to implement. One other thing that these longest living societies have in common is that until recent years (sadly, worldly goods are now much more easily transported and available) there was very little consumption of refined sugars and processed foods.

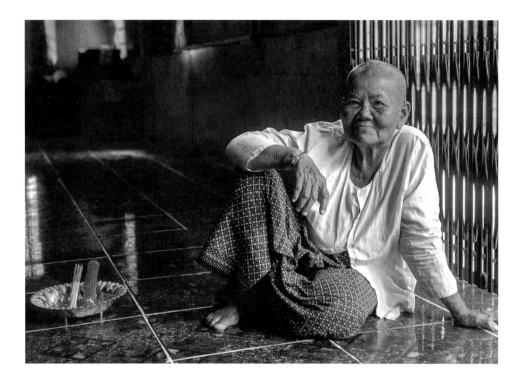

I think what we need to do is to 'be the change', and once we are the change, and people see us making a difference, they will follow suit. We have to love ourselves enough to love the food that is going to nourish us. The toughest opponent here though is in your head. Why don't we stop whining and complaining about how tired we are, how depressed we are, how sick we feel, how much we want to succeed, how much more energy we require ... and just crack on! Do you want to create a confident, strong, and capable you? Everything in your life is a reflection of the choices you have made, whether you like it or not. If you want a different result, make a different choice. It doesn't take generations to change, it takes just minutes.

Six out of ten people in the Western world have cancer. Young people are getting sicker, younger. More babies have brain cancer and leukaemia than ever before, and heart attacks are happening every second somewhere in the world. The fat contained in animal foods (meat) loves heavy metals and holds onto deadly chemicals, the very things that are causing challenges to our bodies and so much disharmony. Today more than 95% of all chronic disease is caused by food choices, toxic food ingredients, lack of nutrition, and sedentary lifestyles. Lack of exercise will kill you, but equally over-exercising can also harm your body if you are not nutritionally supported. You see, all disease comes from an element of free radical damage. We can repair and get antioxidants from salads, greens, raw fruits, and vegetables, juice and smoothies. (I am talking proper healthy vegetable-based juices and smoothies.)

In the Western world one in five breakfasts is purchased from fast food restaurants. For starters we don't need vast amounts of food for breakfast. When we sleep we are fasting and this is the best chance your body has to repair and renew all your luscious cells that want so desperately to keep you well. Whatever you have for breakfast must be nutritious and health-giving because that is going to set you up for the day. Take the average Western diet. Breakfast consists of milk and sugar-laden cereal, cups of coffee, sticky pancakes, bacon and eggs, and a ton of toast. Or if you are going down the fast food route, beige stodge. It is a recipe for disaster, not success and vibrancy. You will wake up groggy, get up and pile in this acidic and quite toxic plate of so-called foods, and your brain will feel foggy, your emotions all over the place or, worse still, deadened.

Have you ever seen the documentary *Super Size Me*? If you haven't, take a look at what this kind of food can do to you. If you want to be a brain-struggling zombie, then fill your boots. Go ahead and see how you feel starting your day this way. My advice would be to wake up and have a health-enhancing tea, or hot water and lemon, followed by a home-made green juice. I can promise you that if you do this your body is going to jump for joy and you will feel the energy rising. If you can go to the gym or do some sporting activity such as running after this little concoction, see the difference in your energy. Then around 10 or 11 a.m. have your breakfast.

In the meal suggestions I will explain more about food choice, but as long as you understand the basic principles that's all that matters. Remember, the more you over-eat, the shorter your lifespan is! Take cholesterol as an example of a health problem. In Westernized parts of the world there have been suggestions that if you are over 50 you no longer have to take a cholesterol test. Why? Because you are simply auto-matically put on statins or similar medications to keep your cholesterol low. What about educating everyone on healthier eating? What about teaching children in every school how to prevent disease so it just becomes the norm? Is it because there is no money in this? Because the drug companies need people to be sick? These types of medications have side effects. They can cause severe muscle pain, liver damage, kidney failure, and even death!

Many people consider the raw food diet to be radical. I am not suggesting for one moment that you transition immediately, or ever completely if that's not what you want. But knowledge, my friends, is power, and once you know these things, it might just be the wake-up call you need to make better choices. The point I am trying to make is this: reversing serious diseases is possible. I have seen it with my very own eyes, and it's magical. The question is would you rather have your chest sawn in half and your heart taken out of your body or would you rather change your diet to prevent that happening? Quite a choice, hey! Look at what so many other species eat. Horses, cows, squirrels, rabbits, gophers, groundhogs, elephants, goats, sheep, antelope, deer, elk, moose, kangaroos, birds and many more just live on a plant-based diet. They are strong and energetic.

Another massive problem we have is a large number of the world's population are losing their memory. This is directly linked to a lack of vitamin B12 and of essential fatty acids in our diets. A few days ago I was writing my newspaper column in a coffee shop in Guildford, on my way back from my London clinic (drinking green tea of course!) and I saw a sweet old couple opposite me doing a crossword. They were loving what they were doing and so engaged with each other. They seemed to get it solved relatively quickly. It was such a coincidence, as this was the very subject I was writing about and there they were, as if to confirm what I wanted to say. If I was an artist (which I can guarantee you I am not, stick men is about as far as I can go!) I would draw them. They both looked old and weathered, but healthy and beautiful at the same time. They had a glow to their skin as if they spent time outdoors and rosy cheeks from the cold. I have no idea if they were husband and wife, as they arrived separately, and they looked really pleased to see each other. He greeted her with a kiss on the cheek and they barely said a word before they sat down and entered into their crossword puzzle-solving. It's almost as if they met just for this very purpose. Maybe without realizing it, they have got it right. When it comes to your brain power, if you don't use it you lose it. It needs training every day. Like every other muscle in your body, it needs to be in constant use and fed the most beneficial foods in order to maintain its full functioning capacity.

The other important thing about absorbing nutrients from your food is that simple act of chewing! Not only does chewing create mindful eating and appreciation for your food, it also helps to mechanically break up your food and stimulates saliva production for lubrication, helping the digestive enzymes to begin working efficiently. The more you chew, the smaller your food particles are and the more nutrients your small intestines can absorb. As 70% of your immune system is in your intestines, this simple act is essential.

The easiest way to get sick is if your digestion is not happy, and it will literally make you feel miserable. So rather than cleaning up the digestion and trying the simple things first, we prescribe antidepressants instead, which just continues the circle of ill health. Why not look at diet or anything else related to health in order to try and get this person back on track instead of throwing some other toxic drug at this epidemic. Let's clean up the diet and see what happens before we go down that route.

It's true that antidepressants can be life-savers. Recently, a very close friend of mine was suffering from severe depression and the medication did help temporarily to dig him out of a very deep hole. But in the long term, it's not the answer. I have clients that come to me and have been on antidepressants for 20 years or more. The side effects can range from sleep problems such as insomnia, headaches and dizziness, tremors, shaking and feeling anxious (ironic), pain, weakness, yawning and feeling tired, loss of appetite, nausea, vomiting and diarrhea, dry mouth, sweating, and hot flushes.

What your cells actually want is oxygen! When you eat sugar, for example, you reduce available oxygen by a third. Even eating fructose from fruits can reduce oxygen if you overdo it. Wheatgrass is the perfect tonic for increasing oxygen in the body. Two ounces of wheat grass, which is a tiny amount, is equivalent to eating 5lbs of green vegetables. The fact is that with the vast majority of the drugs you take there is a chance you might experience some kind of side effect. Try breathing, exercise, and food before you try medication. All raw food, especially greens, contains oxygen. Once you cook your food, just be aware that in most cases the nutrients start to diminish. The fragrance that you smell when you cook your food is actually the oxygen leaving the food. The rawer the food you eat, the greater your enzyme activity is, and the less chance you have of developing serious disease. Even diseases like multiple sclerosis can be helped by this way of living.

Let's look at milk as another good example of what we need to understand. 100 calories of watercress give us roughly 800 mg of calcium. 100 calories of collards give us 548 mg of calcium. Spinach 450 mg and rocket 1300 mg of calcium. That's a lot! One glass of milk on average contains about 300 mg of calcium. According to Dr T Colin Campbell, an American biochemist who specializes in the effect of nutrition on long-term health, casein, which makes up nearly 87% of cow's milk protein, is carcinogenic. More research is being done constantly on all areas of nutrition, and I am sure you can do your own too and come to your own conclusions. But I wanted to point out that all is not as it seems, and advertisers can lead us into a very false sense of security. It's about looking beyond and having an open mind to the world around you.

In relation to feeding cattle, redirecting even some of the grain used to feed them could potentially nourish every hungry mouth on the planet, not to mention the water usage: 1 lb of steak takes around 2400 gallons of water to produce. Take a look at the *Cowspiracy* documentary to find out more about how the meat and dairy industry cause a colossal amount of environmental issues too, so let's not just blame global warming on car, plane, and train emissions.

As far as sugar is concerned, if you want a healthier alternative, stevia is a natural substitute that might just help wean you off the white stuff, but don't just use it as a switch from one sweet thing to another. The point is to reduce your consumption. Cancer, diabetes, arthritis, insomnia, osteoporosis, and heart disease all like sugar very much. In fact those life-altering diseases can suck the life and vitality from you after you've had your fill of sweets for the day. Sugar weakens the bacteria in the gut and efficiently helps to destroy your immune system. Eating a plant-based diet will regulate your blood sugar levels and feed your body with the best substances you can imagine. The higher the quality of foods, the less disease you have the potential of developing. Treat your body with the tender loving care that it deserves. *There is NO specific diet that will do what healthy eating does*. Stop the radical diets and get engaged to your lifestyle. This is not just a two-second wonder, these are permanent lifestyle choices.

You can be the richest billionaire on the planet, but it's not going to save you. Look at Steve Jobs. On his deathbed he wished he had done things differently – spending more time with his loved ones was one thing he was clear about. There was no doubt that the man was a genius and changed our technical world, but it couldn't buy him health in the end. You're prepared to pay out for health insurance, and spend money on all sorts of vices, yet people tell me all the time that eating healthily costs a lot. Actually, it really doesn't have to, but how can you put a price on your health anyway when you are so prepared to invest in other things such as cars, houses, gym memberships, alcohol, shoes, handbags, cigarettes! Whatever you spend your money on, there is no investment like your health. How about making green juice, superfood and vegetables your health insurance instead?

ADVICE: In my opinion your best six doctors are:

1. Sunshine
2. Water
3. Rest
4. Air
5. Exercise
6. Diet

If it really is important to you, you will find a way. If not, you will find an excuse.

The four things you will gain from engaging in better lifestyle choices are:

1. **Balanced hormones** – this will protect you from premature ageing and disease.

2. **Increased oxygen** – which will feed your cells and protect you from premature ageing and disease.

3. **Increased phytochemicals from better food choices** – to feed your cells and protect you from premature ageing and disease.

4. **Increased enzymes** – from better food choices, creating the spark of life which will help every cellular function in your body and to protect you from premature ageing and disease.

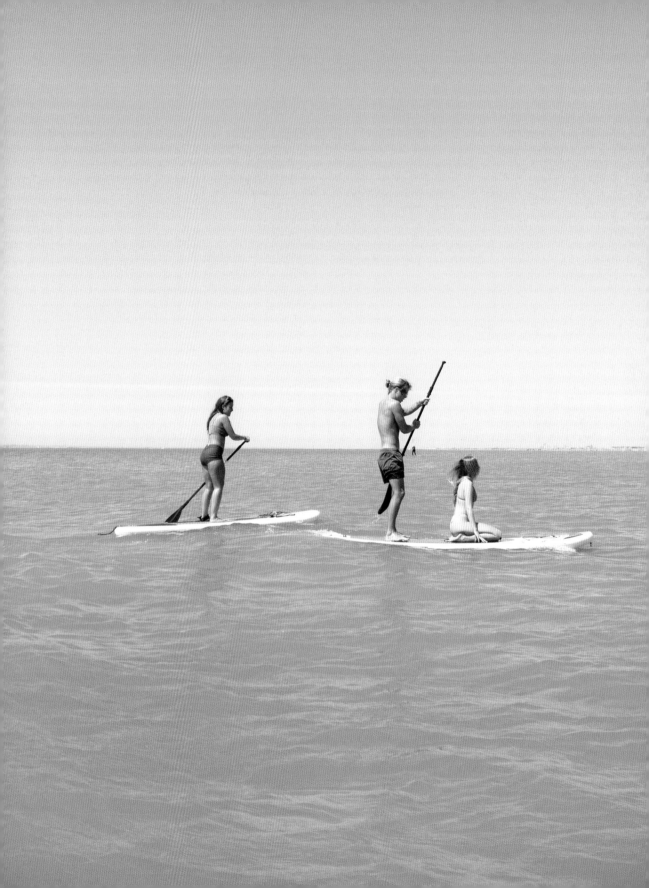

CHAPTER 8

THE TOP EIGHT FOODS TO INCLUDE IN YOUR DAILY DIET

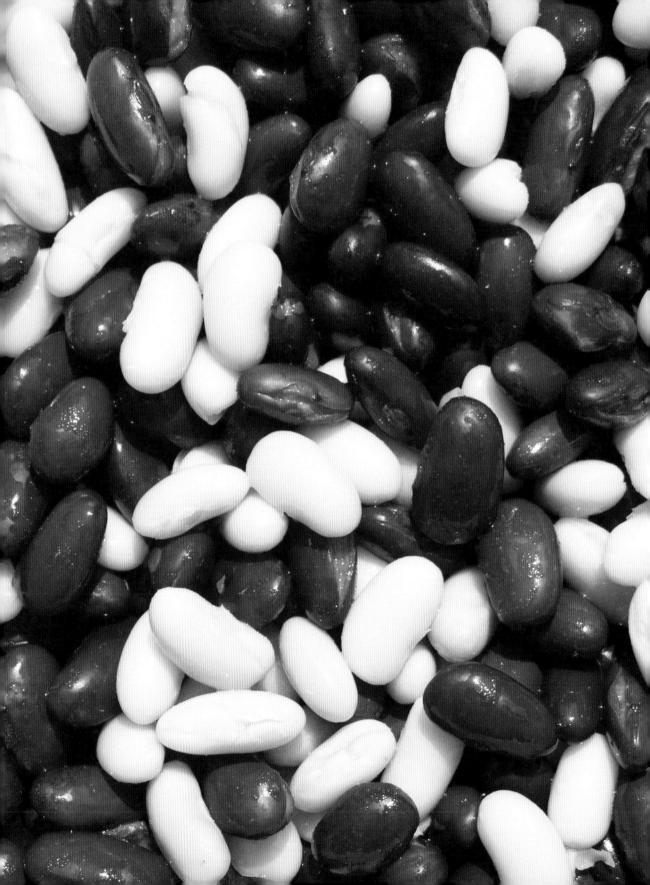

have talked so much about all the things we shouldn't have in our diets, so let's get down to business. What foods should we include?

To maintain energy, good bowel health, great digestion, and to keep disease at bay, we must concentrate on eating as many of certain food types as we can in one day. There are good reasons for this, as you will see.

Beans

Beans including black beans, butter beans, cannellini beans, peas, kidney beans, haricot beans, pinto beans, split peas, lentils, and chickpeas. Some of the top cancer researchers from across the globe have summarized that some of the best things we can include in our diets every single day, in fact not just every day but at every meal, are whole grains and beans. Most of your plate should be covered with vegetables and whole grains, with the remainder of your plate being beans. Why? Because they are loaded with protein, iron, and zinc, and they have a high fibre, potassium, and folate content. They are free of cholesterol and naturally low in saturated fat and sodium.

These little beauties are not to be underestimated. They reduce our risk of depression, stroke, and colon cancer. They not only help to prevent breast cancer but increase survival rates too. And they help you to stay lean and slim, lower your blood pressure, regulate blood sugar, balance insulin levels, and help you to feel full and satisfied. You can disguise beans in many dishes you can eat throughout the day such as houmous, or pea soup. Make these fresh and you have yourself a tasty health-enhancing snack full of goodness. Just quarter of a cup of houmous, or half a cup of pea soup for each meal is enough for your daily intake. You can prevent prediabetes by eating these little gems and stave off heart disease and osteoporosis too. Why wouldn't you?

Cruciferous Vegetables

Cruciferous vegetables include bok choy, broccoli, broccoli sprouts, watercress, turnips, radishes, Brussels sprouts, cabbage, cauliflower, collard greens, and kale. Cruciferous vegetables are the most powerful source of antioxidants and including an array of these in your daily diet will offer you outstanding protection from many diseases. They not only help detoxify the liver by boosting enzymes, they also boost our intestinal immune cells to help us fight against pathogens and toxins. They are considered one of the top two vegetable families that help cancer prevention, alongside the allium family, which includes garlic and onions. The intake of these vegetables helps reduce bladder, prostate, and lung cancers, and keeps your brain and body strong and fit. Interestingly, kale may be more beneficial cooked than raw. To maximize levels of sulforaphane, which helps to protect our brain and eyesight, as well as preventing a variety of cancers, it is recommended to either pre-chop the vegetables at least 40 minutes ahead of cooking or add a pinch of mustard powder during the cooking process. The rest of these vegetables however can be eaten either raw or lightly steamed. Personally, I prefer the flavour and feeling I get after I have eaten them raw, and still like to chuck raw kale in my daily smoothies.

Greens, Greens, and More Greens

Greens are the healthiest vegetables in the world! Any dark green leafy vegetables are considered the most effective when it comes to the body absorbing nutrients. Greens such as kale, broccoli, spinach, romaine lettuce, peas, Brussels sprouts, beet leaves, collards, cabbage, watercress, swiss chard, and rocket. They are inexpensive and highly beneficial, being packed with important and powerful nutrients crucial for good health. Eating whole plants outweighs any benefits from taking supplements, and even as little as one serving per month reduces the risk of glaucoma by 69%. The lutein and zeaxanthin found in greens protect against cataracts and macular degeneration too and these green gods can massively improve your skin, by reducing wrinkles and protecting you from free radical DNA damage. They can also improve your dental health as well as supporting and boosting your immune system.

Amazingly, research has suggested that two or more daily servings of greens can help clear the human papillomavirus, which has been clearly linked to certain cancers. Greens will also reduce the risk of breast cancer, kidney cancer, and lymphoma, as well as providing overall cancer protection for many other specific types. This is the answer you are looking for when you ask 'Where am I going to get my calcium from?' The solution is greens! The calcium in dark green leafy vegetables is more effectively absorbed by the body than anything you can absorb from cow's milk. The potassium helps prevent heart attacks and strokes and is fantastic at reducing inflammation. They provide a high level of antioxidants, and an array of minerals vital for good heath such as iron, zinc, and magnesium. The high levels of folate in greens seem to be more effective than supplements and can help reduce depression too, because of the healthy whole food fats found in greens. You can get similar results from nuts and seeds.

A plant-based diet tends to be more alkalizing which is a substantially healthier environment for your body and is more effective at preventing disease. Nitrates are high in greens, and it is this that is believed to help prevent against the risk of heart disease and high blood pressure. Greens help protect your muscle mass and improve your physical ability and athletic performance. In abundance they can help reduce your risk of gout and kidney stones. Personally, I think the most effective way to get greens into your body in high volume daily is to put them in your smoothie. This way you have an array of vegetables and goodness giving your body the greatest fighting chance for outstanding health.

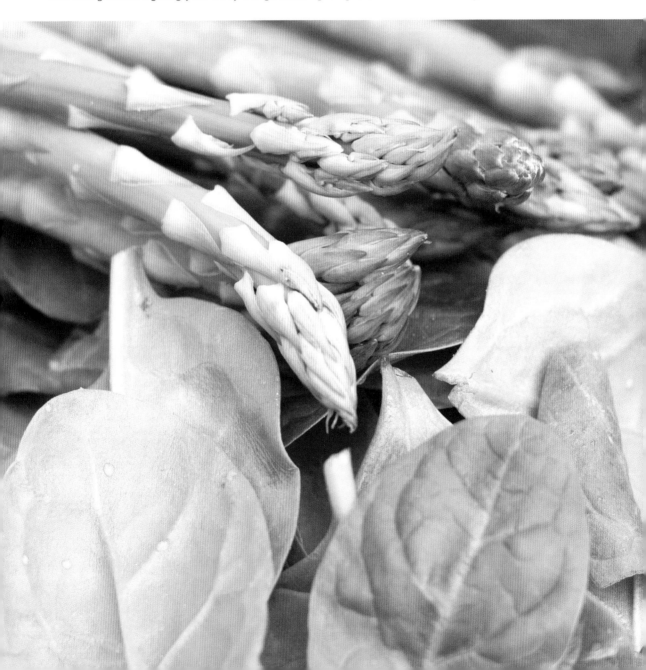

Berries

The best health-promoting berry fruits are acai berries, barberries, blackberries, blueberries, cherries, cranberries, goji berries, and raspberries. These are delicious and healthy fruits, mainly because they are so colourful and contain antioxidant pigments. It is the colour that provides the antioxidants. For example, red onions have more antioxidants than white, red apples have more than green, red cabbage has more than green, and red grapes have more than green ones. Do you see the pattern? There are other fruits that come a close second, such as apples, plums, dates, clementines, dried apricots, avocados, dried figs, bananas, pears, and pomegranates, although berries average nearly 10 times more antioxidants than other fruits and vegetables. And they have over 50 times more than any animal-based food. Berries are said to double the count of natural killer cells, rapidly improving the body's immune system and helping to protect from viruses and cancerous cells. They also improve memory and reduce oxidative stress in anyone participating in long endurance exercise. They help protect the liver and keep your skin looking young and fresh. Because they are high in fibre and low in calories, they help to keep your arteries clean and healthy, making them fantastic for heart health. They are rich in minerals and vitamins, including vitamin C, iron, calcium, and vitamin A. What's not to love?

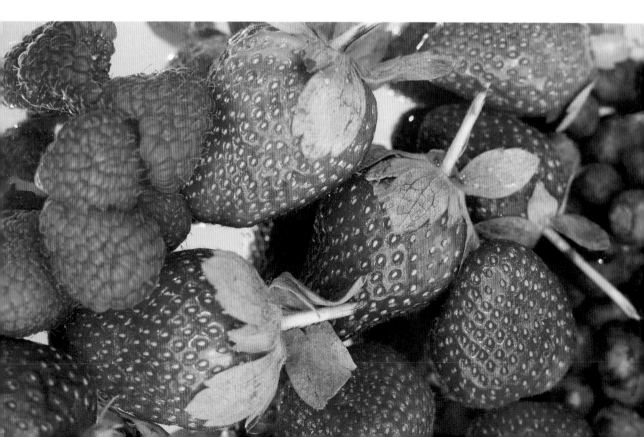

Whole Grains

Whole grains such as oats, whole wheat, brown rice and quinoa are a massive asset to any health seeker's diet. People who eat the most wholegrains have significantly less narrowing of both the coronary arteries that feed the heart, and the carotid arteries that feed the brain. Atherosclerotic plaque in the arteries is a leading killer, so by eating whole grains and whole foods (vegetables, fruits, whole beans) you could possibly reverse life-threatening conditions completely. Eating whole grains helps to reduce the risk of strokes, heart disease, high blood pressure, type 2 diabetes, obesity, and cancer. Increasing our daily consumption could potentially save the lives of over a million people around the world every year. One and a half cupfuls per day is about right, so divide that between three meals and there you have it … your little bundle of health.

Nuts and Seeds

These little treasures of nature are incredibly powerful when it comes to nutrition. The combination of phytonutrients and antioxidants put these high on the list of priorities to include every day. They are an excellent source of healthier fats. The fat from nuts and seeds will help with the absorption of certain phytonutrients and is therefore much more likely to be better for cardio risk factors than, say, the fat from olive oil. Seeds are a source of arginine which will help boost fat burning. They also contain high levels of magnesium and tryptophan, which is a fantastic stress reliever. Many people suffering from digestive conditions such as diverticulitis have been warned to stay away from nuts and seeds, but the latest research is suggesting that sufferers eating these foods actually had lower rates of inflammation.

If you are including flax or chia seeds in your daily regime, it can help prevent diabetes, cardiovascular disease, menstrual and breast pain, and joint pain and can reduce the risk of depression. Flax seeds, fenugreek seeds, and mustard seeds are potential sources of melatonin, which help to control your sleep and wake cycles – vital for good health. Sesame seeds are a great source of phytosterols, which help reduce excess cholesterol. Dried pomegranate seeds are very high in antioxidants, and many other seeds can be sprouted for amazing health benefits, broccoli being the best for hormone-related conditions. You don't need a massive amount of nuts every day, just a palmful will do. The healthiest nuts in my opinion are pecans, walnuts, hazelnuts, pistachios, and almonds.

Herbs and Spices

You need herbs and spices in abundance in everything you cook. Why? Because they contain a wide array of antioxidants, minerals, and vitamins, and they improve the nutritional density of any meal. Let's call it a 'food upgrade' without any calories. These flavoursome wonders rank even higher in antioxidant activity than fruits and vegetables, and most of them tend to have unique medicinal qualities and are a dose of anti-inflammatory magic. The common thread to many diseases, as already mentioned, is inflammation in the body. So being liberal in your use of herbs and spices is a simple way of keeping your health in check. They are often inexpensive and have such an impact on your health that you will soon realize you cannot live without them. They have been used in medicine for thousands of years and can help alleviate the symptoms of, or prevent, diseases such as cancer, arthritis, Alzheimer's, depression, and anxiety. The most common herbs and spices that will have the biggest benefits for your body and should be used daily are: garlic, ginger, turmeric, rosemary, cloves, cinnamon, oregano, coriander, cloves, saffron, lemon balm, marjoram, and black pepper.

Health-enhancing Beverages

Green tea has been proven over the years to help ward off numerous health issues, such as lung cancer and heart disease. It is believed to stop the malignant transformation of cultured breast cells and has even been thought to be helpful when it comes to preventing dental cavities. It's a low-calorie brain booster and a great health protector, so including two to four cups daily will improve your levels of protection. Other teas have health benefits too, such as tulsi tea, dandelion, and hibiscus which are all said to increase the antioxidant levels in the bloodstream within a very short space of time. Some studies suggest that in as little as one hour improvements can be seen. Matcha tea is another excellent protector. You could potentially drink up to 10 cups of a variety of teas per day and the more varied the better. Beet juice is another favourite of mine. It has so many beneficial effects on the body, such as improving both mental and physical stamina. It also improves your blood circulation, memory, concentration, libido and sexual function, as well as increasing your energy levels and it gives you a fantastic amount of minerals and vitamins. Green smoothies and juices are also great options to keep your energy high and your nutrients flowing.

CHAPTER 9

TOP POWER SUPERFOODS FOR THE UNSTOPPABLE YOU!

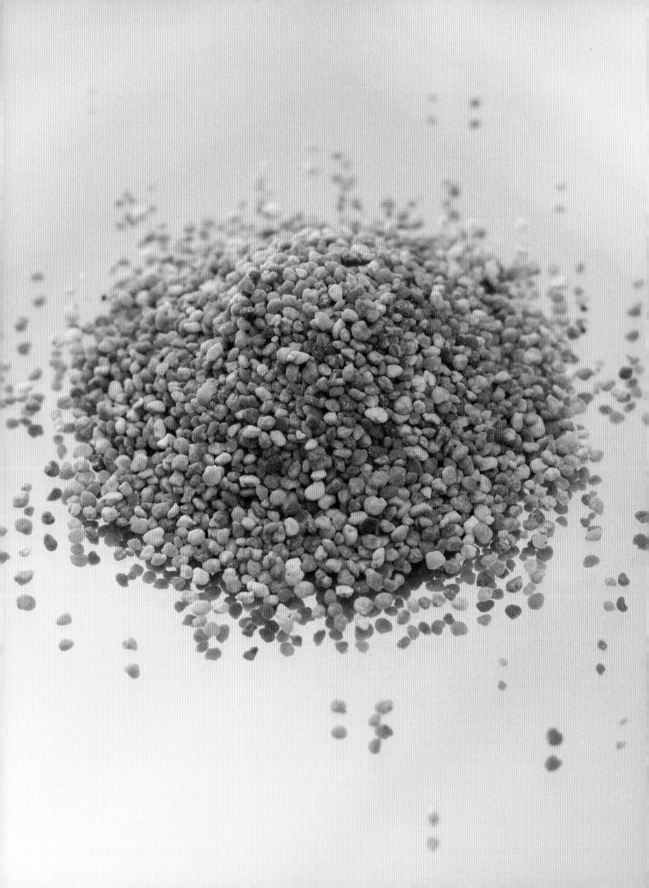

Everyone's looking for a quick fix or a magic pill that does it all. A pill that keeps you slim, helps you to stay young forever, gives you more brain power, better stamina, more energy, and more focus. While I cannot offer you one magic pill, I can introduce you to powder superfoods that could potentially rock your world. When I first started using superfoods many years ago, I couldn't believe how different they made me feel. We don't have all the nutrients in the plants and the soil that we used to have, so this is the answer to topping up the tank. Every day we need to bombard our bodies with life-enhancing substances, and in my experience, not only as a nutritionist, but personally, with myself and my family using superfoods, this has to be the best thing I have ever experienced with regard to nutrition. I could live on smoothies lavished with superfoods every day, and nothing else.

Nutritionally, an array of superfoods has all that you need to keep you alive and kicking, without the stress of digesting heavy meals that you really don't need. When you eat clean, energy-enhancing whole foods and superfoods, it gives you such a feeling of lightness and sustained vigour. When I don't have them in my diet I miss them. I don't take them all at the same time, but gauge how I feel from week to week, sometimes day to day, and use what I feel is best at the time. You can, however, choose to use as many as you like in one smoothie. They do not contraindicate each other and will only enhance your energy. That's the beauty of them: once you learn and understand the purpose of each, you can play with them to suit your needs. As they are a food substance, your body is able to digest and utilize the nutrients in the best possible way. In other words, we can absorb all the goodness and nutrients, giving our body maximum power.

I prefer them to manufactured vitamins and minerals, for the simple reason that they are as nature intended them to be, and in my experience most people respond well to them. They are much more readily available now than they were even 10 years ago, and you can find many of my favourites in good health stores and even some supermarkets. So, what exactly does 'superfood' mean? It is the term that refers to a food that contains health-promoting properties, therefore reducing the risk of disease by improving any aspect of physical or emotional health. They may be unusually high in antioxidants, vitamins, and nutrients. I always prefer to take superfoods in their original state, so I tend to prefer powders over pills. Also, when you buy anything in powder form you are buying by weight and can control exactly how much you spend and how much you take daily.

The superfoods I describe here are in no particular order. I love them all, and each and every one has a positive part to play in enhancing our daily health.

Chlorella

This single-celled green algae cultivated in freshwater ponds has been around for billions of years and is amazing! The water it is grown in is oxygenated, then filtered for purity, and has been a key health ingredient in places like Japan and other Far Eastern countries forever. It's one of the healthiest, most potent foods in existence, not only for humans, but for livestock all over the world too. It's a rich source of chlorophyll, which helps the body to cleanse the blood, cells, and organs from a build-up of toxins such as heavy metals, poisons, and medications. So essentially when you consume chlorella, it works like a little Pacman, clearing out all the baddies from your fabulous body. Adding this incredibly powerful superfood to your diet increases your red blood cell count, which creates more oxygen to promote healing.

Chlorella causes the friendly bacteria in the gut to multiply at four times the normal rate, which is vital for good health. This is a superfood that provides us with excellent nutrition so we can heal ourselves and restore wellness within the body. Being 60% protein in the form of amino acids makes it far superior to meat, fish, and eggs because of the way our bodies can absorb goodness. It also contains crucial life-enhancing enzymes and an array of vitamins. When taking this superfood, in my opinion, you do not need to take any other multivitamins as this will provide you with everything you require.

It's a superior digestive aid that enhances the intake of nutrients, clears up bad breath, keeps the delicate pH of the blood in balance, and improves muscular strength so much that if athletes use it they risk less injury. Chlorella energizes each and every cell by assisting in growth and repair, and it also strengthens internal organs and dramatically boosts the immune system. Adults and children can take it as a preventative strengthening superfood. This superfood has been used in health clinics to treat many types of cancer. It's also beneficial for diseases such as Alzheimer's and dementia, helps lower cholesterol and blood pressure, and contains several compounds that are considered to be antioxidants, such as vitamin C, beta-carotene, lycopene, and lutein.

How much should you take? You can read all sorts of different suggested dosages on the internet, but in my experience as a maintenance health dose, I would say 1–2 teaspoons per day is ample.

Bee Pollen

This is a brain-enhancing, sexy, exuberant, powerhouse, natural multivitamin! This is as nature intended. Being an enzyme-enhancing mineral and energy-blasting superfood you can give it to your bambinos, your granny, your mother, your father, the Queen … oh, and, of course, yourself. It's amazing, it's brilliant! It doesn't come from the bees, it comes from flowers. The bees collect it, bind it with enzymes and bring it back to the hives. It's not strictly vegan, but can be sourced ethically where they just collect the pollen that is brushed off the bee's legs as they enter the hive, leaving some food for them. We all live on the same planet and it's possible to share in a peaceful way without destruction.

Bee pollen has a range of benefits that will blow your mind. It possesses anti-ageing properties, as well as stimulating cell renewal and rejuvenating the skin. It is renowned for increasing longevity and has a good reputation for its anti-cancer properties and reducing tumours. It helps protect against radiation and can help combat the side effects of chemotherapy. It is fantastic for improving fertility, by stimulating the ovaries and improving the libido, mainly because it's packed to the rafters with 96 nutrient elements. It contains all 22 amino acids, and is approximately 40% protein, making it a very sustainable food. It's massively high in B vitamins (including the best dietary source of B6 and a reputed source of B12) and vitamin C, the best dietary source of rutin, a glucoside, which strengthens the capillary system, and one of the richest sources of carotenoids and bioflavonoids.

It is high in zinc, which is great for prostate problems, and has significant amounts of potassium, calcium, phosphorus, magnesium, silicon, manganese, sulphur, selenium, and iron. It is rich in lecithin so has a great synergy when taken with flax oil, as it allows oils to be easily integrated into the cell membrane. It is also an excellent source of phenylalanine which regulates natural appetite. This gem of a superfood has been used to treat Crohn's, colitis, and peptic ulcers, and is a powerful natural antibiotic. Many people use this in conjunction with weight loss programmes as it stabilizes blood sugar levels, and it is superb for treating anaemia and cardiovascular issues, as it can normalize cholesterol and balance the metabolism.

How much should you take? For general health benefits start with half a teaspoon, per day building up to a tablespoon or more if necessary. For allergies and hay fever, source local pollen and begin with just a few grains under the tongue and then build up to a teaspoon. Take at least six weeks before hay fever season starts to build up a resistance (it works like a homeopathic remedy).

Yummy factor: It's pleasant! Quite waxy, but sweet and easy on the palate. Take either with other foods (adds a slight sweetness), especially good in smoothies, or take on its own for a quick boost of 'buzzy' energy.

Contraindications/precautions: Goes rancid easily so you must keep in a sealed jar in the fridge. May cause digestive discomfort because it is so rich in enzymes, so take very little initially. May cause a mild allergic response such as itchy skin or tingly lips in which case the person may need to detox more first or gradually build up resistance.

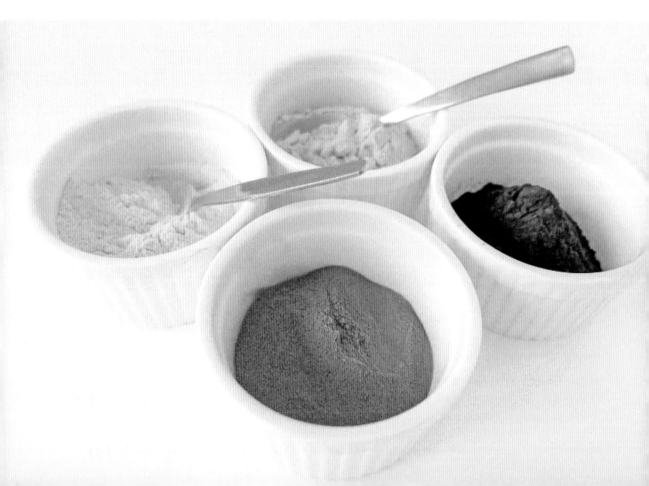

Spirulina

Spirulina is right up there with the world's most popular and nourishing superfoods, spirulina is an organism that grows in both fresh and salt water. It is grown in environmentally controlled ponds especially constructed for this purpose. It is a blue/green algae just like chlorella, but I would use them for different purposes. It was eaten by the ancient Aztecs as they knew what was good for them, especially their beauty and their health, and this amazing product was bought back to life when NASA proposed that it was so nutrient rich it would be suitable to be grown in space for use by astronauts. I use this product with my clients for its high protein content as it supplies 20 times more complete protein than soybean and meat, and it's rich in enzymes, chlorophyll, magnesium, potassium, calcium and phosphorous.

It is well known for its incredible B vitamin content. That makes it a great product for people with fast-paced lives, excessive stress, and lots of activity as it supports energy levels and helps massively with muscle repair and general stamina. It contains essential fatty acids that help to regulate hormones and keep your brain highly powered and is rich in beta carotene which helps to overcome eye problems caused by vitamin A deficiency. Spirulina works fantastically well as a great sidekick for chlorella, as the two combined are incredibly powerful, offering different nutritional elements. Spirulina contains a high level of antioxidants, contributing to removing toxins, which improves energy, fertility, digestion, elimination, memory, mental clarity, depression, weight control, blood pressure, arthritis, PMS, eczema, skin health, bone strength and also helps to reduce inflammation.

How much should you take? Keep it simple and use in the same way as chlorella. Just 1–2 teaspoons a day of this gorgeous green stuff is going to help you so much. If you know you have heavy fitness training programmes, or lots of corporate events, or something taxing coming your way, add a little more into the mix. You will get to know the balance that works for you, but this is a fantastic product to take every day to support your body optimally.

> **Yummy factor:** Slightly more potent than chlorella, but honestly the cleaner your diet, the more you get used to this flavour. Tastes a little seaweedy! Just disguise in your smoothies or coconut water. If you feel like you are catching a cold or fever, just add more and it will disappear in no time.

> **Contraindications/precautions:** In large doses can cause headaches, allergic reactions, and sweating. People with an allergy to seafood, seaweed, and other sea vegetables should probably avoid spirulina.

Baobab

I love this white powder so much! Honestly, if you try it every day for one week you will start to notice a significant difference. It's rich in vitamin C (said to be 10 times more than an orange) high in calcium (twice the calcium of a glass of milk) high in potassium, (four times that of one banana), and high in magnesium (five times more than an avocado). It is being used in beauty products now for promoting skin elasticity and is said to maintain your healthy youthful glow. It's an edible fruit that has been known forever for its health properties and is grown in Africa, Australia, and the Middle East. To get the powder as we know it, it is taken from its natural environment and dried, removing the seeds and being ground into powder that can be added to food products.

Classed as a citrus fruit, and containing antimicrobial, antiviral, antioxidant, and anti-inflammatory properties, this product is not one to be missed. It is said to be the superfood that can treat 'any disease'. That's a bold statement, but as it has had success in treating malaria, tuberculosis, fever, microbial infections, anaemia, toothache, and dysentery, I think we can safely say this precious fruit can benefit your health and boost your immune system in a pretty powerful way. It can improve your digestive system, helps with general hydration of the skin, and seriously supports your endocrine health. With its high mineral content and high fibre and protein, this can be a real asset to your daily intake. It's great for body builders as it supports the muscles and is a powerful anti-inflammatory superfood, which helps to alleviate muscle and joint pain – it can match the power of many medicinal painkillers.

How much should you take? 2–3 teaspoons per day. You can safely take more of it you have a hardcore lifestyle.

> **Yummy factor:**   Pleasant! Doesn't taste of too much, and is easily mixed in water, smoothies, juice, or sprinkled on food.

> **Contraindications/precautions:**   None, as far as I am aware. Not enough studies have been carried out yet, but as it's been used for centuries I would think it is pretty safe. Obviously if you are pregnant or breastfeeding, I would suggest doing your own research to make sure you are happy.

Pine Pollen

Be careful with this one. It's not necessarily the superfood that I would suggest for everyone, but it is a potent healing, nutrient-dense superfood that is slightly off the radar as far as superfoods are concerned. With over 200 bioactive nutrients, minerals, and vitamins in high concentration, pine pollen is extremely effective. Is it one of the few substances on earth that has the ability to stimulate measurable testosterone and hormone production. Pine pollen is literally the pollen from pine trees and is a type of seed. It contains the fundamental nutrients and essence necessary to grow a towering 100-foot-tall pine tree that can live for hundreds of years.

Not surprisingly, it contains rare nutrients that can do much the same as the human body does. It promotes rapid growth, healing, and rejuvenation. In Asia, pine pollen is known as a Jing-enhancing herb, which translates to 'life force'. I would use it with my clients mainly for weakness, burnout, stress, exhaustion, and sexual imbalances such as erectile disfunction, low libido, and infertility. It contains hundreds of nutrients, such as B vitamins, amino acids, vitamin D3, and DNA-repairing fragments such as nucleic acids as well as numerous antioxidants. For me, the best quality is its ability to harmonize and rejuvenate the endocrine system and the remarkably clever adaption that occurs naturally in your body to whatever conditions are present, and whichever hormone you need more of, be it testosterone, oestrogen, or progesterone, it can balance you perfectly.

How much should you take? there are many different formats, but I still love the powder best. Stick to a low dose of one teaspoon per day and see what results you get. This is a little more potent, so take with caution.

> **Yummy factor:** Pleasant to taste! Add to smoothies, juice, or water.

> **Contraindications/precautions:** DO NOT give to male adolescents under 20 years old due to their already budding hormones. Supplementing any bio-identical hormone at puberty or younger is discouraged as this can affect the body's ability to produce that hormone normally later on in life. If you know you are allergic to bees, you may have a reaction to pine pollen. Just take with caution in the beginning until your body gets used to it. Check with your GP if you are taking any hormone-related medication.

Beetroot Powder

If you have bad circulation or high blood pressure then look no further. Or if you suffer from anaemia, indigestion, constipation, or dandruff this powder, made from ground up raw beetroot, is magnificent. Brilliant for cardiovascular health and reducing cholesterol by increasing the levels of good cholesterol in the body. Fibre also strips excess LDL (low density lipoprotein – the so-called bad cholesterol) from veins and arteries to help rapidly reduce unwanted cholesterol. It also cuts down your risk of stroke due to being especially rich in potassium. This red powerhouse is fabulous for pregnant women, because of the high level of B vitamin folate, which helps with the development of the baby's spinal column and can also help with general fertility.

Beetroot contains betacyanin, something that helps counteract the growth of cancerous cells and they can inhibit cell mutations. Beetroot also assists in slowing down tumour development in the lungs, colon, and skin. Maintaining a healthy liver can also be helped by this wonder powder as it is good at preventing and reducing the fat in this organ. Because of its high vitamin C content it's a great support to the lungs and has been reported to reduce symptoms of asthma. But maybe the best benefit of all is the boost to your libido due to the significant levels of boron, a mineral that has been shown to increase the production of sex hormones. They not only help to increase your sexual appetite, but also contribute to improving sperm mobility and increase fertility.

Beetroot powder is the most impressive brain food, helping improve both Alzheimer's and other forms of dementia, but can also support general memory enhancing by protecting the hippocampus from damage. This is the part of the brain devoted to memory and learning. How about achieving a spot-free, glowing looking skin too? Well, this is the product for you as it's an excellent source of iron and anti-inflammatory properties. It not only tightens your skin, but reduces dark spots, including bags under your eyes, and blemishes due to its being a natural blood purifier.

How much should you take? Put 2–3 teaspoons per day in your smoothie, coconut water, or water.

> **Yummy factor:** Delicious! It adds colour and a delicate flavour to your smoothies. Anything red is going to have massive benefits to your health! Especially your heart.

> **Contraindications/precautions:** Taken in large quantities it can cause allergic reactions, such as rashes, hives, and itching. And it can cause kidney stones in rare circumstances.

Wheatgrass

Taking wheatgrass in powdered form might be simpler than juicing your own, as it's easier to just pop in your smoothies, but of course the real deal would be better. But we are after quickness here, and it's still around 79 per cent as effective as the juice you could squeeze yourself. Wheatgrass is an energizer for the mind and the body, and the vitality you gain from this is unbelievable. Two ounces of fresh juice equals three pounds of vegetables in vitamins and minerals! Wheatgrass is super nutritious, containing 90 out of the 102 vitamins, minerals, and nutrients that you need in a day. High in vitamins A, B, C, E, and K as well as calcium, chlorine, iron, magnesium, phosphorous, potassium, sodium, sulphur, zinc, and 22 amino acids, it is safe to say it's a good healthy choice! It's a whole meal and complete protein, high in enzymes and chlorophyll, which helps to build healthy blood, improves circulation, reduces toxicity, and stimulates healthy tissue cell growth.

Ann Wigmore was a very famous lady from Lithuania, who believed she healed her own body from cancer using wheatgrass juice and other raw vitamin and enzyme-enhancing foods in the 1950s. She went on to live another 35 years of health and well-being and spent the rest of her life teaching and educating people on natural health and optimum healing. Her use of wheatgrass was a key dietary component in her own healing, and many people have claimed the same experiences since. She maintained that it drained the lymphatic system, which carries many of the toxins out of the body cells, and when disease occurs, in the form of inflammation (arthritis, eczema, etc.) there is a natural build-up of mucus in the lymphatic system in that area. Wheatgrass will break down the mucus and allow it to clear. It also supplies iron, which helps to cleanse the blood and prevent anaemia.

How much should you take? 1–2 teaspoons daily is good. Or 1–4 ounces if juicing.

> **Yummy factor:** Tastes like grass! Not too bad if you are OK with grass! But very worth it for the excellent health benefits.

> **Contraindications/precautions:** Taking too much can cause nausea, constipation, and loss of appetite.

Maca

This is a powerful superfood traditionally used to enhance fertility and sex drive, but honestly it's so much more. It's a cruciferous vegetable related to broccoli, cauliflower, cabbage, and kale and has a long history of medicinal use in Peru. It is the root that is the edible part and the fact that it is able to grow at high altitude gives it its strength and power when ingested by humans! I use it for people who are under intense stress, or those enduring hardcore activites such as marathons or ironman competitions because it gives robust and lasting energy. It helps you to feel strong, grounded, and calm, and much more in control of life. The plant itself has a very high frost tolerance, so it helps to maintain body temperature.

This beautiful natural herb helps reduce feelings of stress, anxiety, trauma, and fatigue and dissolves the patterns that are creating disease. It contains a high level of antioxidants, relieving chronic fatigue syndrome by balancing the adrenal glands, which results in better energy levels. It is a fabulous hormone supporter too, and is known for improving fertility, in both men and women, as it contains so many minerals, including magnesium, potassium, zinc, iron, phosphorous, selenium, and manganese. It also alleviates symptoms of the menopause due to the natural decline in oestrogen such as hot flushes, vaginal dryness, mood swings, sleep issues, and irritability. It contains omega 3 and plant extracts that can boost physical performance and helps the body to fight issues such as eczema and other skin complaints. It contains glucosinates which have anti-cancer properties and inhibit tumour growth and can be very helpful in the reduction of an enlarged prostate.

How much should you take? Take with caution as maca can sometimes wipe people out if they are already exhausted. I would suggest half a teaspoon to begin with for one week, then increase to a maintenance dose of 1–2 teaspoons in smoothies. It is best not to take directly off the spoon as it can stick to the roof of your mouth and this isn't too pleasant!

Yummy factor: Quite an earthy flavour, but palatable.

Contraindications/precautions: Do not take if you have thyroid issues because it contains goitrogens, substances that may interfere with the thyroid's normal function.

Pea Protein

Take pea protein for a great physique! Most people think the only way to get a lean body is with a protein-rich diet. And we get our protein through meat! Right? Wrong! When you think of muscle builders and people who work out all the time with lean, mean fighting-machine bodies, the last food that springs to mind is a lovely little green round garden pea! But pea protein is not just for body builders. People in all walks of life can benefit, for extra protein strength and stamina. The main reason that pea protein powder, sold in most health shops and even supermarkets, is gaining in popularity is because it is rich in branched chain amino acids (BCAAs). These are protein compounds that have been shown to delay fatigue during and after exercise.

It is fantastic, because the amount of BCAAs in pea protein comes close to those found in milk and eggs, but as more and more people become allergic, or have reactions or intolerances to these food types, this offers a safe and amazing alternative that will do you the power of good. It is promoted for people taking part in physical activity and healthy body building, but actually it's suitable for many other things. For example, pea protein also contains arginine, an amino acid shown to enhance immunity. It also fights erectile dysfunction and can help improve fertility. The lysine content in peas supports the body in absorbing calcium, helping to maintain strong bones, and, since peas are a plant, it's a protein source that's lower on the food chain and in line with the general shift towards a plant-based alkaline enhancing diet.

So, if you are feeling like you need a little muscle power, whether you are 18 or 80, maybe a little pea protein is the answer.

How much should you take? Simply pop 1–2 teaspoons of powder into your drink, smoothie, or juice!

> **Yummy factor:** Tastes good.

> **Contraindications/precautions:** Pea protein can be high in sodium so if you are on a restricted diet you may need to watch the amount you take in.

E3Live

This is a wonder of all superfoods. This powerful liquid algae, which you can knock back like a shot of tequila, is bursting at the seams with wellness. It has to be kept frozen and the best way to defrost it in order to drink, is to remove some from your freezer every morning as soon as you wake up, let it defrost for a few hours and then enjoy two shots during your day, putting the rest back in the freezer to repeat again, like groundhog day, the next day.

So what is it? E3Live is 100% Aphanizomenon flos-aquae (AFA) blue-green algae, which is a certified organic wild harvested nutrient-dense aqua botanical considered by renowned health authorities to be one of nature's most beneficial superfoods. It supports your immune system, your endocrine system, and your nervous system, protects your heart, and improves your gut health. This magnificent, almost tropical-looking product provides a staggering 65 vitamins, minerals, essential fatty acids, and amino acids and is a rich source of chlorophyll. Studies are fast proving that eating a small amount of this blue-green algae every day supports the body in protecting against cancer and viral infections, as it helps to produce natural killer cells. It also contributes to the reduction of inflammation, is filled to the brim with antioxidants, and contains high levels of protein, vitamins, and minerals. It boosts energy levels and can be an amazing kickstart for weight loss. It also supports the mind/body balance due to its incredible nutrient-rich content.

> **Yummy factor:** Well, I don't want to lie to you, it's quite pond-like, but as you need so little (a shot glass full twice a day – preferably one in the morning and one mid-afternoon) then my suggestion would be to just neck it … quickly, followed by a little tasty chaser of coconut water or fresh juice! Like all these things, the more you take, the more you will learn to love them, especially when you feel and see the health-enhancing benefits!

> **Contraindications/precautions:** Take initially with caution. If you take too much too quickly it can cause stomach pains. This is usually due to the high level of good bacteria that it can produce. It can also cause detox symptoms such as headaches because of the highly cleansing effect it has on the body. It is generally considered a safe product for all ages.

Chia Seeds

If you haven't tried them yet I would highly recommend you get a packet of chia seeds for that special ingredient to give you lasting energy and brainpower. They don't look pretty, or taste of much, but when this little black bundle of power is soaked, these chias are going to give you a boost to your well-being that you will never want to live without. Chia seeds are incredible and give us lasting energy, helping to maintain our blood sugar levels so we feel like we have the drive and vitality to take us happily through the day.

These black seeds originate from the central valleys of Mexico and come from a plant source that is reputed to have been eaten as a staple food by the Aztecs. Chia seeds are regarded as one of the most important crops to the Aztecs, next to maize and beans. For the best results you will need to soak them overnight in water (one table-spoon in a cup of water will do). If you forget to do this, do not despair! As soon as you get up in the morning, nip into the kitchen and pop them in to soak for 10 to 15 minutes. You know when they are ready to eat because they get gloopy and become surrounded in a gel-like liquid. These health-enhancing seeds are beneficial for everyone, including children, the elderly, athletes, dieters, teenagers, or high-powered business executives. These little gems are one of the most powerful, functional, and nutritious superfoods in the world and because they are relatively tasteless, you can add them to all your favourite dips, salads, and sauces and without ever destroying or disturbing the flavours you love.

What will chia seeds do for your health? Chia seeds regulate and balance your blood sugar levels, which is vital for properly functioning hormones and essential for protecting just about every organ in your body. They also lower your risk of diabetes and give you a constant flow of energy. Chia seeds are a dieter's dream as the gel surrounding the seed once soaked is very low in calories and it helps to retain electrolytes in the body fluids, which in turn keeps your heart happy. They are a brainpower food and being a complete protein, enhance stamina, endurance, and strength. Containing a wonderful balance of vitamins, minerals, and antioxidants they can help prevent free radical damage in the body. By weight, chia seeds have more calcium than whole milk and contain an impressive amount of magnesium and boron. Your digestive system will thank you for adding these to your diet as they help to keep everything flowing and hydrated, including the colon and the intestines, making sure all foods passes through with ease. They are also the richest plant source of the essential omega 3.

> **Yummy factor:**   They taste of very little and the texture is like frogspawn! Have I sold them to you yet? Ha ha! They are very inoffensive little seeds that are highly worth integrating into your daily regime. I personally put a tablespoon in my smoothie every day and I would suggest you do the same.

> **Contraindications/precautions:**   Eating too many could interfere with medication, such as blood pressure tablets and insulin, but only because it helps to positively affect both, so you may need to adjust your medication. Not such a bad side effect.

Evening Primrose Oil

Many people associate evening primrose oil with females who have hormone imbalances, but don't neglect the many other things this beauty-enhancing oil is so good at treating. In fact, it is so versatile that I think everyone should take it every day, male and female. If you think about how each and every cell in our body works, we need a good protective but permeable membrane around each cell to allow the good stuff in and the toxins out. Evening primrose oil is fantastic at maintaining a healthy cell, as well as many other things. The oil is from the seed of the evening primrose plant, giving great results for skin disorders such as eczema, psoriasis, and acne, and is extremely effective at treating many other conditions.

When the weather gets colder a lot of people get inflammatory joint pain such as rheumatoid arthritis. The results for this type of pain are fantastic, as are the results for

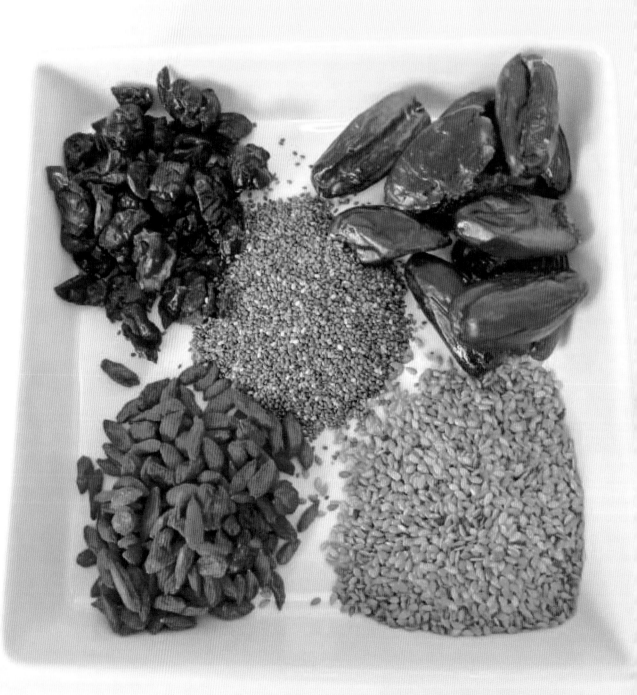

weak bones (osteoporosis), Raynaud's syndrome, multiple sclerosis (MS), cancer, high cholesterol, heart disease, alcoholism, Alzheimer's disease, and schizophrenia. Evening primrose oil is known to help patients with chronic fatigue syndrome (CFS), asthma, and nerve damage related to diabetes. Research shows huge improvements in children's disorders such as hyperactivity and attention deficit hyperactivity disorder (ADHD).

Evening primrose can play a big part in the treatment of obesity and weight loss, whooping cough, and gastrointestinal disorders including ulcerative colitis, irritable bowel syndrome, and peptic ulcer disease. Put the antacids away and reach for some essential fatty acids instead. No nasty side effects and while you are at it, you may see your whole body functioning better, plus your skin will look amazing. Honestly, why wouldn't you? Women have been using evening primrose oil forever, in pregnancy for preventing high blood pressure (pre-eclampsia), or even for starting or shortening labour, and/or preventing late deliveries, but its most classic use is for premenstrual syndrome (PMS), breast pain, endometriosis, and symptoms of menopause such as hot flushes. But men: don't be put off. You can use this too! Don't forget it is an essential fatty acid. Which means it's essential for everyone!

Yummy factor: Tastes of nothing really. It's obviously oily and best taken in your green smoothie or it can be taken direct off the spoon. I would suggest a tablespoon per day as a maintenance dose, and I would also suggest you always buy in a liquid format and not pills. The reason for this is that you get more for your buck and have no gel capsule to digest that could potentially add toxins into your body.

Contraindications/precautions: Always balance omega 6 oils (such as evening primrose oil) with plenty of omega 3 (such as chia seeds) because the two complement each other and we need both!

Colloidal Silver

I have a special love for this antibacterial and antiviral spray that you simply cannot live without. Every household should have it! My niece went off travelling in Africa after doing her A-levels and I gave her a bottle of colloidal silver. It turns out that she used it on everyone for every cut, bruise, sore throat, infection, etc. that she came across. She is a science kind of girl and needs evidence for anything I suggest. Many things we have discussed over the years she thinks are nuts! Colloidal silver, on the other hand, is backed by scientific evidence that it works. It is a health supplement that is created by immersing tiny particles of silver in a colloidal base solution … and it works.

The latest unbelievable finding of this 'wonder' product is that it is helping people with HIV/AIDS and showing positive findings for many patients. It is also fantastic at helping to ward off other serious health ailments such as herpes and cancer. I, for one, have suffered with cold sores/mouth herpes all my life. In the past, every time I had a big event coming up I used to worry that a big blister would just appear through fear! I tried many over-the-counter medications and creams and none of them really seemed to work. Of course, you need to boost your immune system in the best possible way, but sometimes if I am travelling tons, have worked long hours, and had very little sleep I can feel that little tingling begin. Since I discovered colloidal silver it is extremely rare that the cold sore/herpes virus would ever manifest into a full-blown blister. I remember going to a wedding in Italy once and my lip was huge. It was massive, and I felt dreadful. That has never happened again. As soon as I feel that tingling sensation, I start to spray like a crazy woman.

You can spray direct into your mouth and on the area of discomfort up to 30 times per day and the reason it works is this: silver is thought to make the immune system more active and effective at fending off disease. It kills bacteria, even killing off super bacteria that hang around after conventional disinfecting agents haven't been successful. Colloidal silver creates an environment that makes it impossible for pathogens to survive or multiply. There are no known disease-causing organisms that can live in the presence of even minute traces of colloidal silver. Bacteria, moulds, yeasts, viruses, and fungi are all killed off within minutes of contact. Parasites are often killed whilst still in their egg stage. So, if you have an infection, cold, influenza, fermentation, or parasitic infestation this could be your saviour!

It has other uses too. People who have burns can use colloidal silver to promote healthy cell growth in order to heal, plus it's also great at reducing the appearance of acne. And it also helps to maintain a healthy digestion because it maximizes the amount of nutrients that the body is able to extract from food. If you ever suffer from gas and bloating, chances are that this is because fermentation has occurred where foods sit in your system for too long. To avoid indigestion and reflux you can spray colloidal silver directly into your mouth.

> **Yummy factor:** Tastes like water and is perfectly pleasant. Always go for clear colour as the particle size affects the colour of the solution and the larger particles produce a darker coloured liquid but are not so easily absorbed by the body.

> **Contraindications/precautions:** If taken in large volumes it can cause discolouration of the skin. It can also cause poor absorption of some medications.

CHAPTER 10

HOW TO EAT EVERY DAY

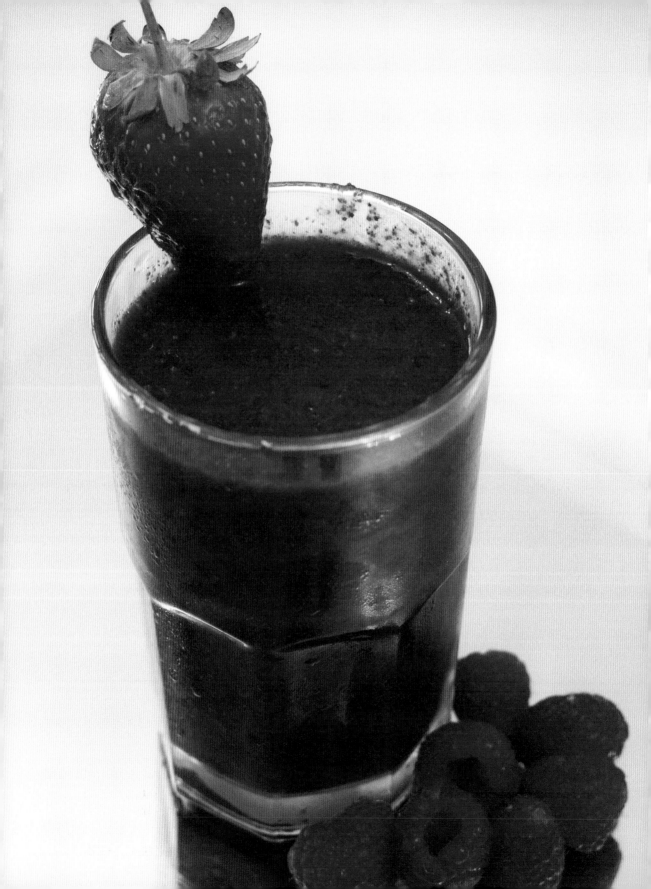

Firstly, before I make my suggestions of how you should eat every day, I think it's important you understand about enzymes. They are extremely important and the food choices you make can dramatically affect them. Enzymes are the spark of life and you need to maintain them in the same way you need to look after your money in your bank account. In the same way you would invest your money wisely, you need to invest wisely with your food choices, or your reserves will run out … it really is that simple.

If you want to stop your hair from going grey, protect your eyesight, keep your hearing tip-top, create healthy digestion, bones, and muscles, and feel like your mind and your body are mentally and physically strong, then listen up.

We have all heard about enzymes, but do we know what they are and what an important role they play in our well-being? All these amazing activities are going on in our bodies every millisecond of the day and we often don't give them a single thought. Enzymes are one of the most interesting and important substances found in nature and make activities possible within each of the 100 trillion cells in our bodies. They are the special added ingredient to allow growth and repair and stabilization within our cells. They are proteins that are organic and work like lightning in our bodies to make things happen. Over 3000 different types of these catalysts have been discovered and identified within our systems and they all have a specific job to do and an alkaline environment is the best and most efficient condition for these little sparks of life to work their magic.

If you look up enzymes in a dictionary you will get a lot of scientific blurb. However, all we really need to know is that they play a crucial role in *all* our chemical processes within the body, including digesting food, transmitting nerve impulses, and making our muscles work. If you think about it that's just about every function we do from blinking and thinking to chewing and pooing!

It is my belief, and I share that belief with many others who have studied this subject for years, that we are all born with a certain constitution. In the same way we are all born into a variety of families, backgrounds, wealth, and health, we are all born with a certain number of enzymes and some naturally have more than others. However, we all have a limited pot! Think of it as a bank account with a million pounds in and throughout your life you start to draw out cash without putting any back. As we get older our cash starts to dwindle, and particularly quickly when we consume what is thought of as the modern, Westernized (acidic) diet such as coffee, milk, tea, chocolate bars, sandwiches, biscuits, processed foods, foods cooked to a frazzle … and the list goes on! The reason we start to become depleted in these enzymes is because these types of foods contain no enzymes at all. So in a way we are robbing our own bank accounts of life-giving enzymes by eating such foods and depleting our systems. Enzymes can only be replenished when we eat raw, living foods which massively aid digestion, which in turn allows us to absorb all the nutrients that we need for the optimal functioning of our delicate but amazing systems.

Enzymes are literally the spark of life! They govern every single function that happens in your body, and every cell needs nurturing and looking after on a daily basis. If you actually stop to think of all the functions we are required to do in a day it's quite mind-blowing!

So, what are the main reasons for eating living foods such as sprouted seeds and raw vegetables?

1. The nutrient value is at its highest when a food is in its natural state.

2. It helps to replenish those all-important enzymes that are *vital* to keep you alive! It's putting money back in the bank account.

When we eat and drink junk it is depleting the account, so as you get older it becomes even more important to look after yourself better. Perhaps that's why we can't quite bounce back so quickly after a drinking session anymore, or why we feel groggy after gorging on pizzas followed by chocolate! Our enzymes are not able to function so well if we eat these acid-forming foods. That's a fact!

It's quite simple really when you think about it! Gorillas in the wild are big, strong, and energetic. Why? They eat their greens … uncooked! Nature is so clever. Raw green vegetables are the most concentrated source of nutrition in any food, with a high amount of minerals such as iron, calcium, potassium, and magnesium. They contain K, C, E, and B vitamins and phytonutrients that protect our cells from pollution, toxins, and damage. So, when your granny said 'Eat your greens', I think she knew what she was talking about!

My first two favourite things are juices and smoothies. I can promise you that if you add these two things into your life you will feel the benefits almost immediately. Not only that, you will see a vast improvement in your skin, hair, and nails and your energy will rise. There are two completely different health reasons why I want you to add these things in and here's why:

Juices

How many of us can realistically eat two to three pounds of vegetables each day? Not many. I know juicing removes the fibre, but it has such great health benefits. I would highly recommend you start juicing if you don't already because it will send your health through the roof. You will have such clean and vibrant energy you won't know what to do with it! Not only that, the whites of your eyes will look clean and glistening and your skin will glow. I know there are mixed feelings amongst the press when it comes to juicing, but if you mostly juice with vegetables (80% vegetables and 20% fruit in each juice) you will not spike your blood sugar and the juice will act like a medicine to your blood – an intravenous drip giving you a wash of magnificent vitamins and minerals like never before. By removing the pulp (the fibre) your body has to do very little to digest. That's why if someone is really sick a juice fast is the best way to heal as it takes very little energy for the body to process and absorb allowing the goodness to go directly into the blood.

As you are drinking and not eating, you are able to take in higher volumes of nutrients, and if you juice twice a day you can add 5–6 different vegetables, including dark greens for your chlorophyll fix. This will keep your blood nice and clean and help nurture each and every organ. Juicing is also very supportive to the good bacteria in your gut, and it helps to keep your immune system fighting fit by adding that extra volume of nutrients. It's far better absorbed by the body than man-made vitamins and minerals, so if you want preventative health this is the way to go. It also helps to detox our bodies and eating foods such as ginger, celery, carrots, lemons, broccoli, apples, and kale helps to lower bad cholesterol; this doesn't overload the system but enhances it.

If I have a juice before a run or a gym workout it has magnificent effects on my energy levels and gives me a much better performance. You can vary your juices so you have an array of vitamins and minerals in each and you can make it in batches giving you enough for three days. Keep in an airtight container in the fridge and there you have it. Your nutritional kick ready to go. Simple! NOTE: buying a more expensive cold press juicer will benefit you in the long run and is worth the investment. It keeps more nutrients in your juice and extracts more juice from your fruits and vegetables, meaning you have to spend less on them. By adding water-based vegetables and fruits, such as cucumbers and watermelon, to your juices you can make larger volumes.

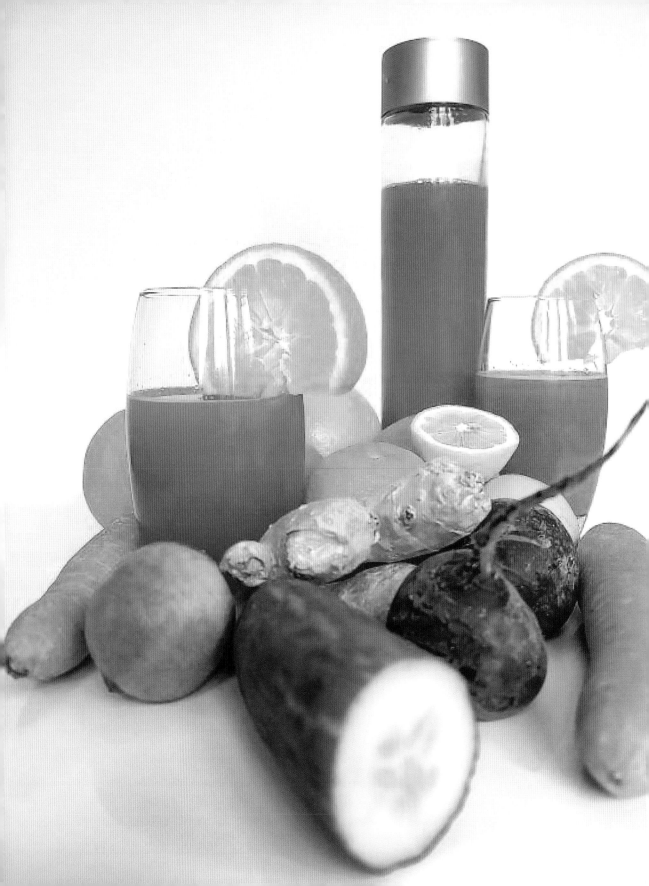

Smoothies

I personally think you should include both juices and smoothies in your daily regime. Smoothies are different from juices as they retain the fibre and you mix them in a blender. I love them because you can add in all your powdered superfoods, and you have an instant blend of utter goodness. Like the juices, this will hugely increase your energy, and topped up with your superfoods, you will feel superhuman after a few days. If you have any digestive issues at all, smoothies are the best way to heal and repair. They will also keep your bowel extremely happy and clean. You may go to the toilet more frequently than normal, but this is good. It's a clear-out, remember I said everything has to flow. Well, this is your nutritional flow and I would highly recommend you do this.

My number one tip is to follow recipes until you get good at making your smoothies delicious. So many people I know just throw in whatever is in the fridge and they taste vile. If they taste vile you will not continue to make them, but if you make them delicious, then all the family can enjoy them. To prevent cancers and other harmful disease, it is recommended that we eat between five and nine portions of fruits and vegetables daily. Smoothies are the best and quickest way to ensure that you are getting plenty more than this. If you want to optimize all the nutrients, this is the way forward. You get a boost of all your vitamins and minerals, strengthen your immune system, and gain extra strength for your bones and muscles. Smoothies will help you to lose or maintain weight, and if you need to gain weight just add extra protein to your shakes in the form of pea, hemp, or flax. It helps to reduce your cholesterol, lower high blood pressure, improve mental focus and clarity, reduce and combat cravings, and is an incredibly effective anti-inflammatory. Basically smoothies are alkalizing, rich in chlorophyll, help with allergies, and can contribute to preventing serious diseases because of the volume of goodness in each and every one!

The number one rule of healthy eating is to be organized. I don't care if you work a trillion hours a week, have 10 kids, and run your own company. Do not tell me you don't have time for healthy eating. It's a fact that we all make the time for things that we want in life and eating healthy food should be no exception. The easiest way to manage a busy life is to plan three days in advance. Whatever you make, prepare, or cook, make enough to stick in the fridge so you can either add to it, or simply take it out and eat or drink.

If you have children, this is a great thing to teach them and they can even help you prepare your weekly juices and foods. The more hands-on they are, the more likely they are to participate, and the earlier you can get them started the better. Being healthy can be so much fun, does not have to cost a fortune, and can be delicious and yummy.

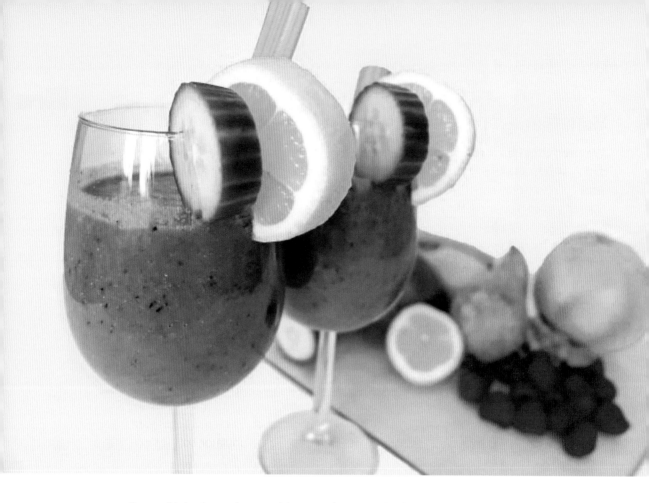

If you think about the nourishment that your body deserves on a daily basis you will have the best mindset to make this work for you and your loved ones. Remember: you might have a predisposition to illness in your family, or a weakness that runs in your genes, but it's your lifestyle choices that will pull the trigger. You are the one putting the foods that *you* choose in your mouth. So the choices are really down to you.

Forget the calories too. If you follow a life-giving diet plan with only whole foods, fruits, and vegetables you will not only gain amazing clarity, have a great body, and more energy than you could ever imagine, you will not have to count calories anymore. You don't want anything other than the foods that are going to supply you with enough nutrients to support your immune system, prevent serious disease, and give you the strength to do all the exciting things you want in your life and the ability to repair and feed your precious and fabulous cells. Life is for thriving and not just surviving, and it's too short for calorie counting! You should be health counting instead!

With our busy lives meal planning is important. Make enough juices, smoothies, salads, soups, etc to last you three days at a time.

Daily Eating Plan

We need to rid the body of toxins each and every day and feed our cells to become super strong and healthy so that all body systems such as the lymphatic, immune, endocrine, skeletal, and nervous systems work smoothly and correctly. This way of living guarantees energy and vitality and allows you to be your natural healthy weight.

When it comes to my meals, feel free to be experimental – after all it's you that's got to eat it.

So, if you like more spice add some, and if you want different vegetables, add them. Use as many fruits and vegetables, herbs and spices in your foods every day as you can to maximize your health!

Wake up: have a cup of warm water, with a cube of ginger and a dash of cayenne pepper. This is a great way to start the day as it continues with your overnight cleansing/fasting and alkalizes the blood, which helps flush toxins from the liver and keeps your lymphatic system very happy. The cayenne pepper is also a slight stimulator, so gives you a similar kick to coffee, but better!

Meditate: even if you can only do five minutes, make time to set your brain up for the day. There are so many guided meditations for free on YouTube there are no excuses at all not to do this.

Dry skin brush: followed by hot and cold showers. This also stimulates the lymphatic system and helps to get rid of toxins. If you work out first thing in the morning you may want to do this after your workout, but either way it's fabulous at keeping you clean inside and out. Always brush towards the heart, up the legs, up the arms, clockwise on the stomach area and down the neck. Then rinse off with two minutes hot water (as hot as you can stand without scalding yourself) and two minutes cold. You can repeat if you wish, and this helps to stimulate your blood circulation and wake you up ready to face the day!

Before you work out: whatever you choose to do, walk, run, cycle, swim, dance etc., I would suggest having your juice. There are three classic examples for you to choose from on pages 150–152. Each one is enough for one day's juice. If you wish to make more for your three days in the fridge, just triple the ingredients and there you have it. I would suggest you use one medium wine glass half full for each juice, and you ideally need two juices per day. One in the morning and one mid-afternoon.

Make your water bottle for the day: it may be a good idea at this point to make up your water. As you are chopping for your juice you may as well cut a few more slices of lemon, lime, cucumber, mint, and ginger for your water bottle. The larger the better so you can sip all day long with your alkaline goodies in. Not only do the fruits and vegetables make the water taste delicious, they add vitamin and mineral goodness to it too. Fabulous! Don't forget to add to a glass container *not* plastic.

Breakfast: start your day with the best foods to keep your body happy. Forget packet cereals, fry-ups and ready-made muffins. Remember your heart needs your help, not your hindrance. See the delicious and nutritious recipes on pages 153–156.

Mid-morning snack (or as a lunch alternative): I would suggest a green smoothie with your added superfoods in to make this the most energizing blended drink you can have. It will enhance your brainpower, help to keep you feeling fresh and alert, and create a body that is truly nourished. See recipes on pages 157–159. I personally would have that as my lunch, but if you are hungry and want something 'solid' then prep some food in advance for lunch. The trick is to feel full after lunch, so you don't reach for the naughty snacks in the afternoon. Eating this way should make you feel really satisfied and energized at the same time.

> ### *Food is not meant to make you tired and lethargic, it is meant to be light and life-giving, so try not to overeat.*

Lunch: having a wrap full of the rainbow salads is probably one of the easiest lunchtime foods you can have. Get a whole grain wrap, or gluten free if you are intolerant, and fill it with radishes, sprouted seeds, green leaves, tomatoes, cucumber, carrots, beets, and asparagus. Alternatively, try one of my tasty salads from pages 160–162. The trick to making a salad filling is to add goodies to it that excite you. Add an array of leaves, such as rocket and watercress, and all colours of the rainbow vegetables. A lovely addition to any salad is watermelon, it's so fresh and gives it an element of sweetness. Or you could add apple, pear, or chopped dates too if you like. Nuts and seeds, spinkled on top, are always filling and grains such as wholegrain rice and couscous can bulk out your salads and keep you full. I always make a salad big enough to last for 3 days in the fridge, so you can have it any time you need to grab something to go to work or eat at home.

If you are a meat eater, or a fish lover, or want to include a bit of haloumi then add some to make it more interesting for you. It's important that the food you eat excites you and you do not need to feel deprived in any way. When you eat in such a pure way you are actually being kind to your body and giving it all the nutrients it needs to fire on all cylinders. Remember most vegetables can be eaten raw and if you start to eat this way you will appreciate the flavours of everything in a completely different way.

Salad dressings: it's all about the dressings! You can make a simple salad taste so much more exciting with the right dressing! Not only that, when you use the correct ingredients it can enhance the goodness of your salad. The simplest dressing is freshly squeezed lemon, some olive oil, and crushed garlic. This makes a tasty and alkalizing dressing. For other options see pages 163–164.

Bowl foods: soups and stews are also a great and easy way to ensure you have healthy meals at the ready. You can make them in a big batch and keep for several days in the fridge and just take out to eat for lunch or your evening meal. They can be light and full of green goodness too and if you live in colder climates, sometimes you need the warmth to soothe you! Use herbs and spices in abundance for extra healing and warmth and add additional things that you love if you wish to experiment. See recipes on pages 165–167.

Green or herbal tea: Switch your milky tea or coffee for a health-enhancing green tea. Or try a herbal tea that could add to your health as mentioned in the health beverage section in Chapter 8.

Mid-afternoon snack: have a second glass of your already prepared smoothie, this will boost your energy and allow you to feel bright and cheery for the whole afternoon. If you get hungry, snack on a protein ball, fruit, or a selection of chopped vegetables that you can dip in humous or an avocado dip. Medjool dates are also a good snack if you are wanting something sweeter.

Around 5 p.m. have your second juice: this will feed your body without using up much effort and if you are going to work out in the evening will help your energy levels immensely.

Evening meals: they should be kept light and, ideally, not be eaten after 8 p.m. Remember the food that goes into your body always needs to feed your system. All evening meals should be small and light, a salad or soup would be great. Always try and eat something raw in the evenings if you can. Even if you want something warmer and cooked, have some salad on a side plate to feed your precious enzymes. See recipes on pages 168–170.

Sweet treats: if you have a sweet tooth and want the occasional chocolate pudding you have to try the one shown on page 171. It's delicious and nutritious and you don't even have to cook it. Or maybe a healthy banana and strawberry ice cream, see page 172. Yes it's good for you and dairy free.

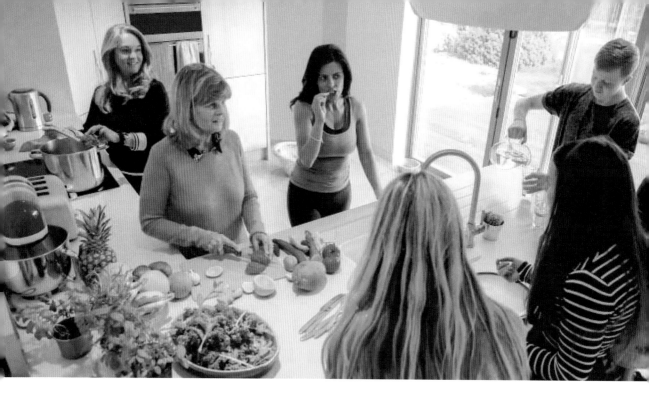

There is so much goodness in all of these foods you could live on them forever. They are full of nourishment that will keep you vibrant and healthy, and alongside your smoothies and juices you are packing a huge nutritional punch every single day.

Evening drinks: herbal teas such as chamomile, lime flower, and peppermint ease the digestion and calm the mind, aiding peaceful sleep.

Have lots of sex: a healthy sex life is good for the heart, especially with someone you really love! It keeps your oestrogen and testosterone levels in balance and helps you to sleep better. It is a massive stress reliever, helps you to burn more calories and lessens your risk of heart attack by 50% if you regularly have sex each week. It makes your immune system stronger, improves your mood, and can even reduce pain. So, if a headache is your excuse, think again! When you orgasm, your oxytocin increases by five times, and this mood-improving endorphin actually relieves aches and pains. Regular sex helps you to live longer because when certain hormones are released during sex, your skin and tissue repairs better, and your blood circulation improves. So not only will frequent sex make you want more sex, because of the elevated hormones, your waistline will thank you and you will feel generally more relaxed, calm, and happy!

Nightly gratitude and evening meditation: be thankful for your day and meditate on positive things for tomorrow.

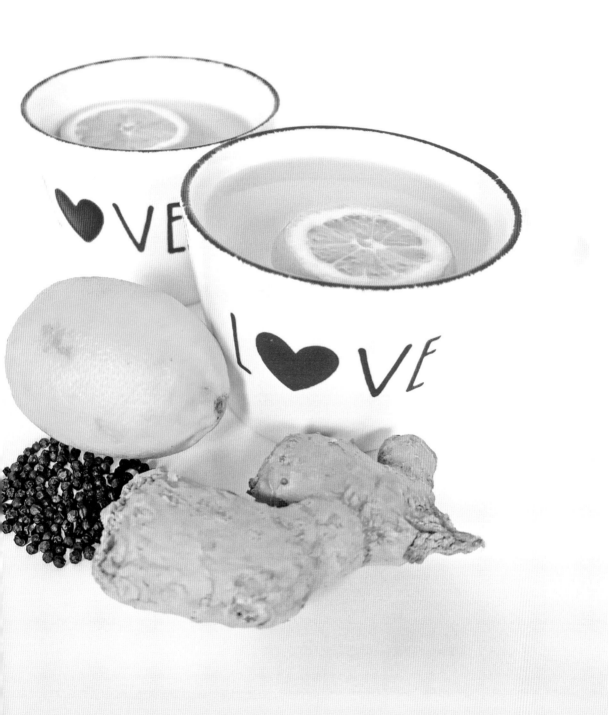

HYDRATION JUICE

This is a super hydrating juice that is going to enhance your natural energy and drench your cells in alkalizing goodness!

INGREDIENTS

½ cucumber

½ watermelon

1 pink grapefruit

2 sticks celery

1 lemon, peeled

handful of spinach

handful of parsley or coriander

5cm fresh ginger

METHOD

Chop all the ingredients and feed them into your juicer. Drink immediately or store in the fridge. Delicious!

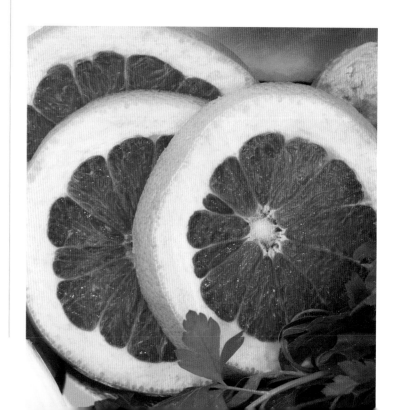

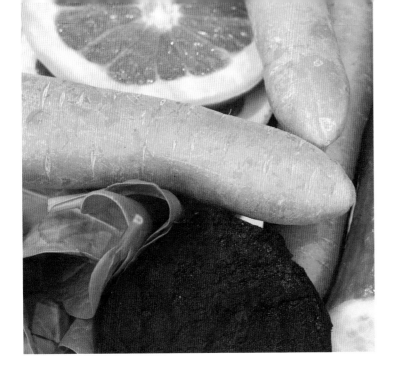

CIRCULATION ENERGY JUICE

If you are getting a cold or feeling run down, you can add one red chilli pepper and a clove of garlic to this juice. Any germs will soon fade away with that potent mix!

INGREDIENTS

3 oranges

2 carrots

1 large sweet potato

1 lime

2 beetroots

½ cucumber

handful of greens such as kale, spinach, or watercress

METHOD

Chop all the ingredients and feed them into your juicer. Drink immediately or store in the fridge. Delicious!

GREEN GOODNESS JUICE

Not only does this taste fresh and delicious it's going to give you such a crazy amount of goodness that your body is going to love you all day.

INGREDIENTS

4 green apples

½ cucumber

1 lime

½ fennel

¼ cup of broccoli

large handful of kale

½ melon (your choice, can be water, galia, yellow)

handful of fresh mint

METHOD

Chop all the ingredients and feed them into your juicer. Drink immediately or store in the fridge. Delicious!

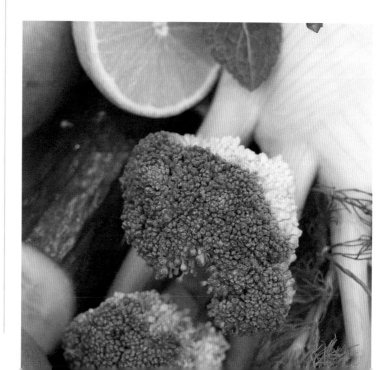

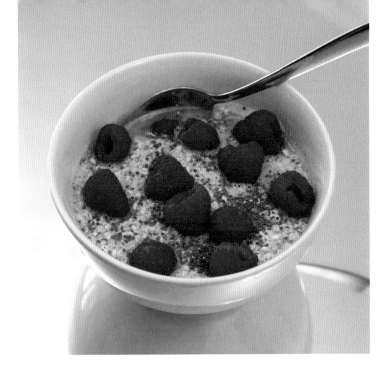

BERRY OVERNIGHT OATS

This has so many good fats, sustainable energy and sweetness from the natural fruits, your brain is going to be firing on all cylinders throughout the day.

INGREDIENTS

½ cup rolled oats

1 tablespoon chia seeds

1 tablespoon ground flaxseeds

½ teaspoon ground cinnamon

1½ cups almond milk or coconut water

2 tablespoons date syrup

1 cup fresh berries

METHOD

Combine all of the ingredients in a medium bowl and mix altogether. Then cover tightly and place in the fridge overnight. It's ready to eat as soon as you need it the next morning.

FRUIT AND NUT BITES

These nutritious bites can be used as a snack in the day, after your morning workout, or simply as your breakfast in the car on the way to work. They can be stored in the fridge and are an easy way to get great goodness into your body.

INGREDIENTS

¼ cup pitted dates

½ cup walnuts and almonds

¾ cup dried cranberries, apricots, or other dried fruit of your choice

½ cup sunflower seeds

2 tablespoons chia seeds or hemp seeds

2 tablespoons ground flaxseeds

½ teaspoon vanilla extract

¼ teaspoon ground cinnamon

METHOD

Soak the pitted dates in hot water for 20 mins then drain. Next add all of the ingredients into a food processor until the mixture is sticky. If you need to add a little water to blend, then you can. Once blended roll the mixture into balls in your hand and put on a plate. Cover the balls and place in the fridge for at least 3 hours. Then they are ready to eat!

You can add a small amount of cacao nibs if you fancy a sweeter treat or if you are transitioning from a higher sugar diet.

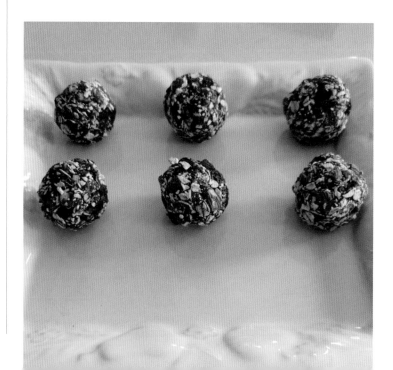

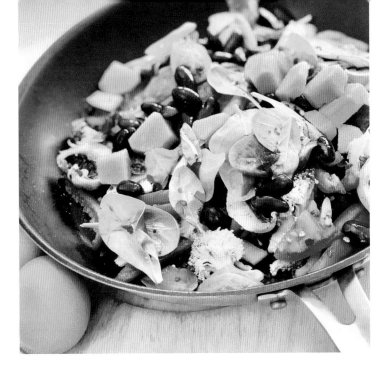

SPICY HEARTY BUBBLE AND SQUEAK

For those of you that wish to start the day with something a little more hearty - this will fill you up and give you sustained energy ad goodness until lunchtime.

INGREDIENTS

1 sweet potato, peeled and chopped

1 small red onion, chopped

1 cup broccoli, chopped

1 red pepper, chopped

½ cup mushrooms, chopped

1 large vine tomato, chopped

1 cup black beans, pre-soaked and ready to cook

handful of spinach or kale

Optional: Cayenne pepper, turmeric, chilli flakes, garlic and ginger

METHOD

Boil the sweet potatoes for 15 mins. Add the sweet potato, onion, broccoli, pepper, mushrooms, tomato and black beans to a frying pan using olive oil or coconut oil for the base. Lightly simmer for 10 mins. If you like it a bit spicy add cayenne pepper, turmeric and chilli flakes to your taste. You can add garlic and ginger too if you like for extra goodness. Then add the spinach or kale for the last 3 mins of cooking. Serve and enjoy.

If there is enough left, you might want to enjoy it for lunch or save it for tomorrow's breakfast. If you eat eggs, you can also add a poached egg or two to this dish for variety.

AVOCADO, TOMATO AND CUCUMBER TOAST

Full of good fats and anti-oxidents you can't go far wrong with this classic breakfast. Delicious and nutritious.

INGREDIENTS

1 whole avocado, sliced

1 large vine tomato, sliced

¼ cucumber, sliced

1–2 slices of sprouted or wholegrain bread, lightly toasted

METHOD

Slice the avocado, tomato and cucumber and add to the lightly toasted sprouted or wholegrain bread. Drizzle with your oil of choice (flax, avocado, evening primrose oil, olive) and sprinkle chilli flakes, pepper, and Himalayan salt.

If you eat eggs you can have one on top, or a tiny amount of goat's cheese or feta. You can be even more creative with this and add olives, greens, nuts, and seeds if you require a more filling breakfast.

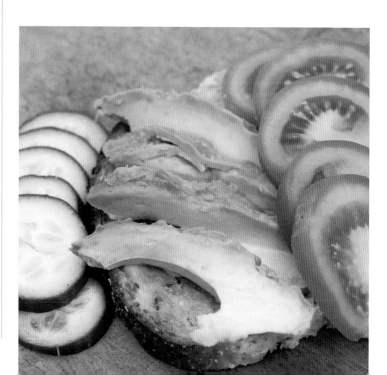

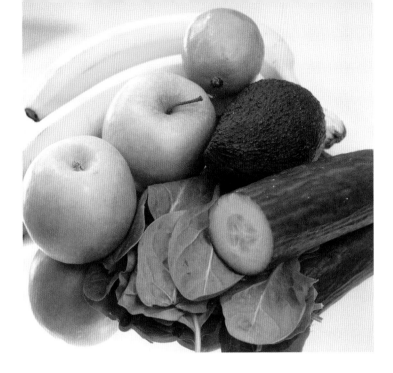

GREEN ENERGY SMOOTHIE

If you want the best start to every day this is the way forward. Your body is going to grow muscles and brain power all in one hit.

INGREDIENTS

2 bananas

1 avocado

½ cucumber

2 green apples

handful of green leaves
(can be kale, spinach,
watercress, chard, mint,
coriander, parsley, etc.)

1 lime, peeled

1 tablespoon chia seeds

1 tablespoon evening
primrose oil

1 teaspoon of each of
your chosen superfood
powders such as
chlorella, spirulina,
maca, baobab, etc.

METHOD

Peel and/or roughly chop the larger ingredients. Place them in a blender and whizz until smooth adding some coconut water or purified water to your mix. Make it thick or runny, depending on what you like. Obviously, the thicker the consistency the more filling this will be.

BERRY BLAST SMOOTHIE

Feeding your body with this delicious smoothie will fill you with antioxidants like never before.

INGREDIENTS

½ cucumber

large handful of berries (can be frozen or fresh)

1 lemon, peeled

1 cup diced pineapple

handful of green leaves

¼ cup fresh mint leaves

1 tablespoon chia seeds

1 tablespoon evening primrose oil

1 teaspoon of each of your chosen superfood powders such as chlorella, spirulina, maca, baobab, etc.

METHOD

Peel and/or roughly chop the larger ingredients. Place them in a blender and whizz until smooth adding some coconut water or purified water to your mix. Make it thick or runny, depending on what you like. Obviously, the thicker the consistency the more filling this will be.

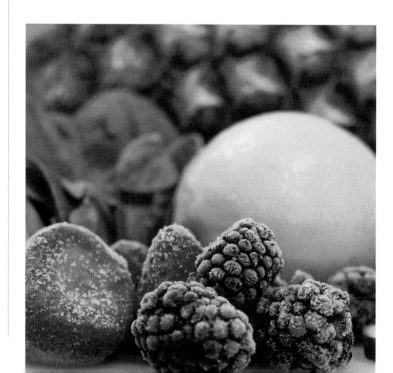

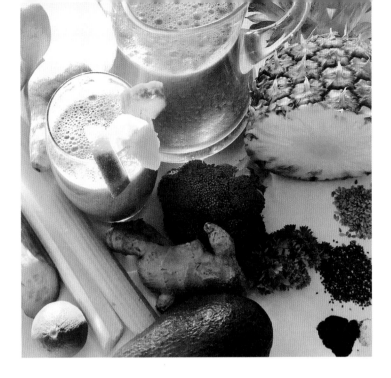

TROPICAL GOODNESS SMOOTHIE

Your digestive enzymes will love you for this delightful smoothie and give you the energy to take you though any busy day.

INGREDIENTS

1 cup diced pineapple
2 pears
1 lime, peeled
3 cm ginger
½ cucumber
2 broccoli florets
2 celery sticks
bunch of parsley
1 avocado
1 tablespoon flax seeds
1 tablespoon chia seeds
1 tablespoon evening
  primrose oil
1 teaspoon of each of
  your chosen superfood
  powders such as
  chlorella, spirulina,
  maca, baobab, etc.

METHOD

Peel and/or roughly chop the larger ingredients. Place them in a blender and whizz until smooth adding some coconut water or purified water to your mix. Make it thick or runny, depending on what you like. Obviously, the thicker the consistency the more filling this will be.

KALE AND MANGO SALAD

The vitamins in this simple salad are insane.

INGREDIENTS

2 cups chopped kale or
baby spinach leaves

1 ripe mango

½ cucumber, finely
chopped

4 radishes

½ cup of sprouted
seeds of your choice

1 ripe avocado

5 baby tomatoes
chopped in half

METHOD

Chop all of the ingredients and add to a salad bowl. Pour over the dressing of your choice. It's as simple as that.

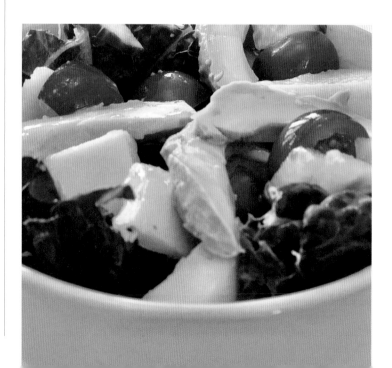

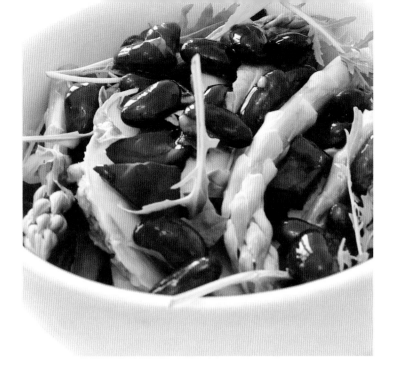

RAINBOW SALAD

Your immune system is going to love you for this one. This array of colour offers a filling fibre packed salad fit for even the hungriest person.

INGREDIENTS

1 red or yellow pepper

½ chopped cucumber

1 small red onion

½ cup red cabbage (raw of course)

1 garlic clove, crushed

1 jalapeno pepper, sliced

1 avocado

5 asparagus spears

handful of green leaves such as watercress, rocket, spinach

Add cooked black beans to this salad for extra fibre and nutritional content.

METHOD

Chop all of the ingredients and add to a salad bowl. Pour over the dressing of your choice. Fast and filling.

NUTTY KALE SALAD

With this many colours your body is going to lap up the minerals and gain some serious strength from these amazing foods.

INGREDIENTS

I bunch kale, raw or lightly steamed

½ cup walnuts and almonds

2 small beetroots, grated

2 carrots, grated

2 vine tomatoes, chopped into small chunks

½ cucumber, finely chopped

small handful of sesame seeds

2 ins ginger, grated

METHOD

Simply chop up all the ingredients, mix together in a bowl and serve.

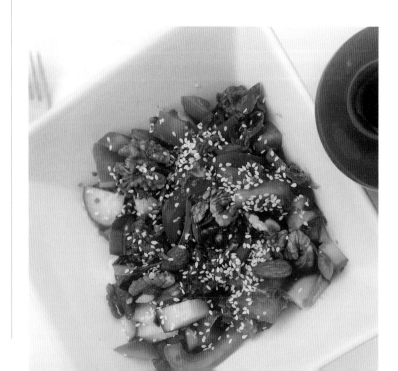

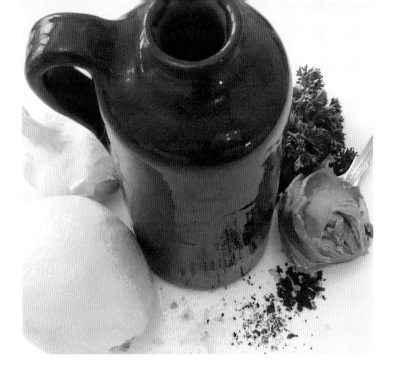

SUPER SALAD DRESSING

INGREDIENTS

2 garlic cloves, crushed

2 tablespoons nutritional yeast

1 tablespoon almond butter

1 tablespoon lemon

1 tablespoon fresh parsley

¼ teaspoon Himalayan salt

¼ teaspoon black pepper

¼ teaspoon chilli flakes (if you don't like too much spice then add less or none at all)

METHOD

Put all of the ingredients in a blender with roughly 120ml of water and blend until smooth.

After blending pour the dressing into a salad jug and keep refrigerated so you can grab some any time you want to spice up your leaves.

GINGER AND GARLIC SALAD DRESSING

INGREDIENTS

2 teaspoons freshly grated ginger

1 garlic clove, crushed

1 tablespoon spring onions

2 teaspoons fresh parsley, finely chopped

2 tablespoons tahini

1 tablespoon rice vinegar

METHOD

Combine all of the ingredients in a blender adding just a teaspoon water until smooth. Transfer the dressing to a salad jug and refrigerate. Spread thinly over any salad to bring it alive.

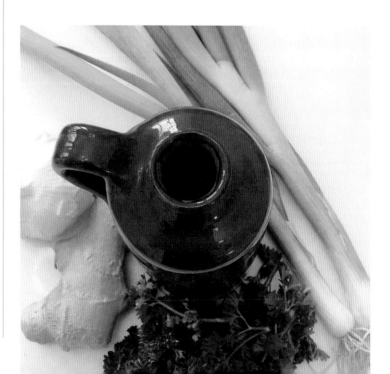

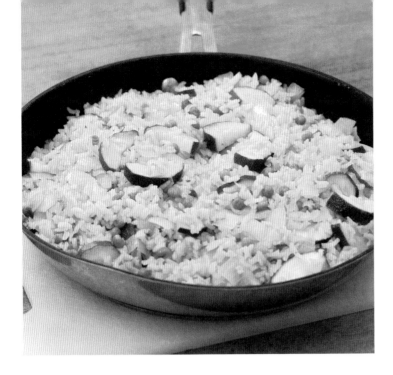

VEGETABLE RICE BOWL

Anywhere. Anytime. This offers so much heathy goodness you can have it for breakfast, lunch or dinner.

INGREDIENTS

¼ cup brown whole grain rice

1 teaspoon olive oil

1 white onion, chopped

1 courgette, chopped

2 cloves garlic, chopped

pinch of Himalayan salt

400ml organic vegetable stock

¾ cup beans, such as haricot or cannellini

½ cup frozen peas

juice of one lemon

2 teaspoons basil pesto (fresh is best)

METHOD

Cook the rice following the packet instructions. Add the olive oil to a separate saucepan over a medium heat. Add in the onion, courgette, and garlic with a pinch of salt and cook until softened. Pour in the stock and the beans. Add the cooked rice, stir in the peas, then add the lemon juice and cook. Ladle into a bowl and garnish with parsley or coriander.

HEARTY VEGETABLE SOUP

This is quick and easy to put together and great to make a larger batch if you want to freeze some for a rainy day. This blast of vitamin rich goodness is going to be great for all the family.

INGREDIENTS

1 red onion

4 cloves garlic

3 celery sticks

2 large vine tomatoes

1 leek

3 sweet potatoes

6 carrots

1 orange pepper

1 tablespoon vegetable bouillon

pinch of Himalayan salt

pinch of black pepper

tablespoon turmeric, fresh or powdered

METHOD

Add all of the ingredients, except the sweet potato, into a pan with a dash of olive oil or coconut oil. Simmer gently and then add your sweet potatoes. Pour boiling water over the potatoes until they are just covered and cook for 15 mins. Whizz to make smooth and serve. You can add a dash of chilli flakes if you like it hot.

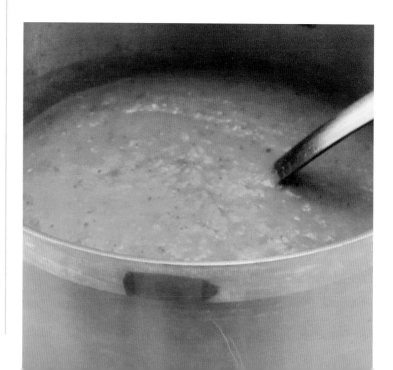

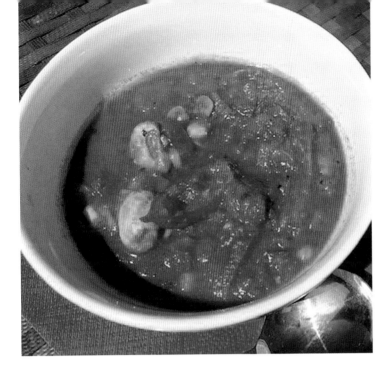

HEALTH-ENHANCING VEGETABLE CHILLI

The spices mean this is a real boost for your metabolism and also a good protector against germs. Having this a few times a week is going to hit the spot.

INGREDIENTS

1 red onion
2 celery sticks
2 cups mushrooms
1 red pepper
2 courgettes
1 hot chilli
3 garlic cloves
4 tablespoons tomato puree
2 teaspoons chilli powder
1 teaspoon fresh or ground turmeric
3 vine tomatoes
2 tins pinto beans
1 cup sweet corn
1 tablespoon of bouillon

METHOD

In a large pan heat up 250ml of water and add 1 tablespoon of bouillon. Add the onion and celery and cook until softened. Then add the mushrooms, pepper, courgettes, chilli, and garlic and cook for 10 mins. Stir in the tomato puree, chilli powder, and turmeric. Add the finely chopped tomatoes, pinto beans, and another half cup of water and the sweet corn. Simmer for 40 mins then serve.

STUFFED SWEET POTATOES

Some sweet goodness for a lunchtime or evening meal.

INGREDIENTS

1 sweet potato

1 cup peas

2 tablespoons fresh chives or spring onions

¼ cup fresh almonds

1 tomato, finely chopped

pinch of ground pepper

pinch of Himalayan salt

METHOD

Bake the sweet potato in the oven for 1 hour. Cook the peas for 5 mins. Once the chives or spring onions and tomato are chopped up, cut the baked potato in half. Scoop out the inner part and mash with the other ingredients. Add the mix back into the potato skin and serve with a dash of balsamic glaze or homemade houmous and olive oil.

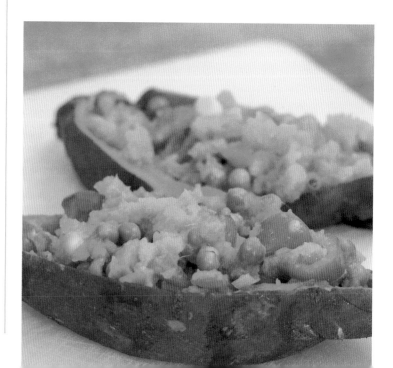

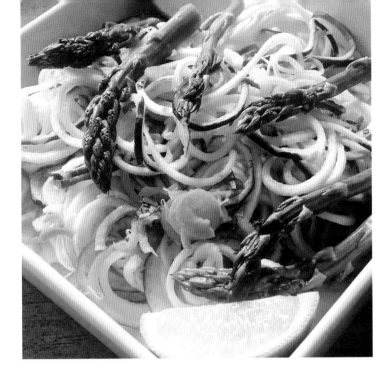

VEGETABLE SPAGHETTI WITH ASPARAGUS

If you don't already have a spiralizer, I would highly recommend that you get one. They are amazing at turning food into creative dishes.

INGREDIENTS

3 courgettes

2 carrots

5 asparagus spears

handful of kale

2 lemons or limes

pinch of Himalayan salt

pinch of ground pepper

3 cloves garlic

olive oil

METHOD

Spiralize your courgettes and carrots until they look like spaghetti and lightly steam them in a pan. Crush your garlic and add to the pan. Add the asparagus and very finely chopped kale to the pan for 2 mins until very warm and lightly cooked. Add the juice of the lemons (or limes) and a dash of salt and pepper with some oil of your choice and mix together and serve.

CHUNKY VEGETABLE TRAY BAKE

This is the easiest dish on the planet. I often prepare this when I get home from work but need to go back out again. It's a great way to ensure we get good food and not too late. You can add pretty much anything you like to this and shove it in the oven.

INGREDIENTS

2 vine tomatoes

1 large sweet potato

¼ cup peas

1 courgette

1 carrot

1 tin beans (red kidney, haricot, etc)

4 broccoli florets

4 cauliflower florets

1 red onion

3cm raw ginger, chopped

4 garlic cloves

METHOD

Chop up the ingredients, add some spices such as chilli flakes, chilli peppers, and some stock and water to the tray so that it covers the veg. Give it a stir and pop in the oven.

When you walk back in the house an hour later you are greeted with the most fabulous smell. Grab from the oven and it's ready to serve. If you want, in the last 10 mins of cooking, you can add some green leaves just to give it that extra nutritional kick. They don't need long at all to cook and are better almost raw, so only give them a few minutes in the oven if you must!

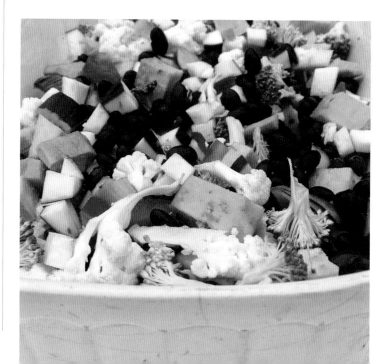

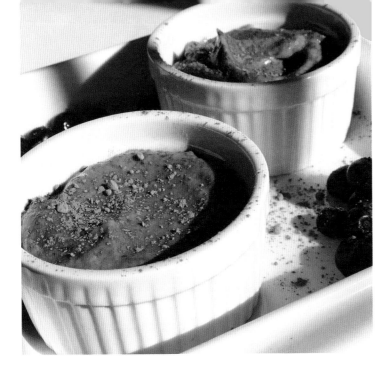

STICKY SWEET TREAT

If you have a sweet tooth then this is the dessert for you. It's super nutritious but very rich, so that will stop you from eating too much. Most of all it's full of goodies that won't cause havoc in your precious body.

INGREDIENTS

1 ripe avocado

2 cups berries

3 tablespoons cacao powder

2 tablespoons almond butter

½ cup date syrup

1 cup almond milk

¼ cup chia seeds

METHOD

Roughly chop the avocado and place in a blender or food processor. Add the berries, cacao powder, almond butter, date syrup, and almond milk and blend until smooth. Then add in the chia seeds and blend until even throughout the mixture. Add to ramekins or small bowls and place in the fridge for at least 6 hours. To make them look pretty when you serve you can add cacao nibs, fresh berries, and flaked nuts if you want.

BANANA AND STRAWBERRY ICE CREAM

It's so lovely to have a couple of spoonfuls of something out of the freezer, especially when you know it's going to do you the power of good.

INGREDIENTS

4 frozen ripe bananas, chopped

2 tablespoons almond butter

1 cup strawberries, chopped

½ teaspoon vanilla extract

METHOD

Mix all of the ingredients in a blender or food processor until smooth. Place in a container and freeze for a couple of hours and it's ready to go. If it becomes too hard just leave to stand before serving. This can be served as an add-on to any delicious fruit salad.

If you make up a mass of fruit salad, with fruits such as apples, pears, berries, pineapple, mangoes, kiwis, etc., a tip for keeping fresh for a few days is to drizzle with lemon juice, which keeps it ready to eat for at least 3 days and also makes is super scrummy!

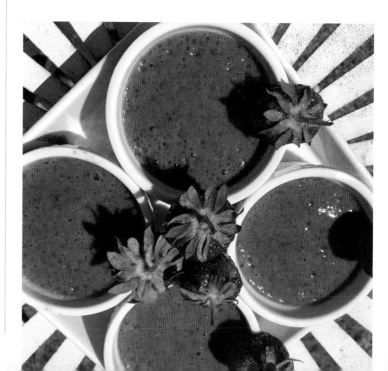

CHAPTER 11

UNDER-STANDING MORE

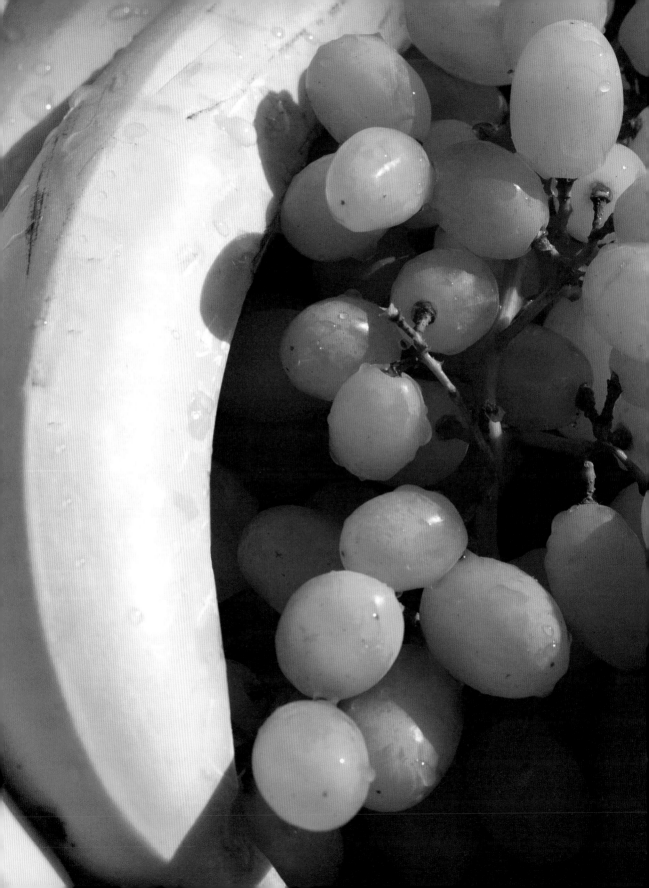

Why Alkalizing and Anti-inflammatory Foods Are the Best Options for Your Health

The most important thing to be aware of is this: it is possible to elevate your mood, energy, and brain power and eliminate pain, discomfort, and inflammation in your body when you eat, live, and move correctly. Whatever you are experiencing right now, such as fatigue and exhaustion, and you require more energy and vitality to succeed in all areas of your life, I can categorically guarantee you that if the majority of your foods are alkalizing and anti-inflammatory you will start to feel more energized and alive.

People all over the world are living with pain that may well be unnecessary. Chronic inflammation is linked to many diseases that I have already discussed. But what about the so-called 'normal' illnesses such as IBS, acid reflux, migraines, hormonal disorders such as polycystic ovaries, infertility, thyroid disfunctions, skin complaints, and inflammation in the form of fibromyalgia, etc. The list of so-called 'common ailments' goes on and on. What is important to understand is that we don't have to resign ourselves to thinking this is a natural part of our life cycle. Whatever your age this does *not* have to be your destiny. I had a friend who visited her doctor recently and he told her the pain she was feeling in her hip was just part of getting older. She's 47! More than likely she needs to visit an osteopath to realign her and then eat some good anti-inflammatory foods, and all will be well in her world.

When you experience inflammation or pain your immune system becomes activated because your body is dealing with something that it does not recognize. Maybe an invading microbe, plant pollen, or foreign chemical. This triggers the 'inflammation' process and the invaders are fought off. Sometimes inflammation persists and then can become your enemy. More often than not it is caused by poor food choices and stressful lifestyles which are accelerating the ageing process and the onset of many health concerns associated with it. When we experience physical symptoms such as swollen joints, psoriasis, immune disorders, fatigue, and digestive issues, there is an internal reaction taking place. The body's immune system has gone into overdrive and this can cause tiredness, aches and pains, and symptoms of discomfort. This is your wake-up call to start making changes in your diet and lifestyle in order to correct the imbalances that are occurring. We regularly see in the press details of the latest wonder cure. However, nothing in my clinical experience is as good as nature intended. Nothing is as good a starting point as looking at our diet and simplifying it. It is unlikely that any improvement will be seen whilst still eating foods that are considered unhealthy. By eliminating the additives that wreak havoc on our bodies and nourishing ourselves with natural foods we give our body the nutrients it needs to begin the healing process.

One key element to getting energized and staying in really good shape is to concentrate on eating alkalizing foods. It is a word that has been very overused in the world of nutrition, but to me it makes perfect sense. It's a very straightforward concept to understand, and I think that once you understand the reasons why something is good for you, it becomes simple to implement into your daily habits. You don't have to be completely rigid with it, but just eating 70% alkalizing foods with every meal will have a dramatic effect on your health. Once this becomes the 'norm' for you the results will be outstanding. You will be rewarded for your efforts with energetic health, a better complexion, and slower ageing. It will also be amazing for reducing the appearance of cellulite, helping with depression and anxiety disorders, and helping or healing just about any other discomfort or ailment you can think of.

The science is short and sweet! Basically, this is why we need alkalizing foods. The pH of the human bloodstream is approximately 7.4. Remember those chemistry lessons looking at the pH scale of 1–14 and testing certain things to see whether they were acid or alkaline? In the same way your body has to balance and regulate your body temperature (a few degrees too high or too low and you are in big trouble) it has to regulate essential fluids such as your blood. Our bodies create acids naturally through our daily bodily functions, and we cleverly have a small alkaline buffering system that works to neutralize these acids. The alkalizing buffers are minerals such as calcium, iron, magnesium, potassium, and sodium and the store of buffers is easily depleted because many people eat and drink very strong acidic foods, such as coffee, burgers, alcohol, bacon, etc. and do very little exercise. On top of that they have a truckload of stress in their lives, smoke, and get very little sleep. This all leads to excess acid build-up within our bodies and can be the perfect breeding ground for disease to manifest.

I describe the acid that builds up in the body as a bonfire that is slowly getting out of control. It gets bigger and bigger until one day it's almost impossible to put out. The reason why some people may be against eating such alkaline foods is because if the body flips too much the other way, we can become too alkaline, and we need a bit of acid to relight our fire. That can affect our digestion and lead to skin irritations. So it's a balance, but I can almost guarantee you one thing. Due to the toxins, pollutions, pesticides, herbicides, stress, alcohol … and life in general, unless you live on a remote island, grow organic fruits and vegetables, meditate daily, and engage only in loving and beautiful relationships you are very unlikely to become too alkaline. In the environments where most of us live this would be almost impossible. In the modern world your body is fighting daily to balance excess acidity, which is why we need such alkalizing foods as they help elimination and increase mineral and vitamin absorption.

Basically, when a body is in an acidic condition, disease or disharmony can occur. The very best way to control disease is to alkalize your system. Simple as it may seem, when you begin eating foods that are alkalizing to your body, symptoms will start to improve, whatever the disease. Please don't take my word for it. Try eating this way and see how you feel.

The rules are basically this – if a food is high in alkaline minerals, including magnesium, potassium, calcium, and sodium, it is likely to be alkalizing to your body. These are foods such as fresh vegetables, salads, leafy greens, omega oils, nuts, seeds, pulses, and whole grains. These are fresh, whole foods and foods with high water content and great nutritional value.

I am sure it comes as no surprise for you to learn that all acidic foods are things that contain sugar, trans fats, yeast, dairy, simple carbohydrates, alcohol, and refined foods. Examples are fizzy drinks, pizzas, chips, cakes, biscuits, microwave meals, crisps, white bread, white pasta, caffeine, cheese, takeaways, fatty meats, ice cream, beers, wines, milky drinks, cream, etc.

Think about your own diet. The average person in a Westernized country consumes over 80% acidic foods each day. What does your diet look like?

The trick is to consume 70% of the alkalizing foods and 30% of the acidic foods every day, preferably at every meal. Give it a go and see what happens to your energy levels, brain power, and emotional well-being!

NOTE: The easiest way to get your alkaline fix is with delicious juices and smoothies. Then eat plenty of salads with luscious little sprouted seeds for that extra mineral and vitamin kick!

These are some examples of highly alkaline foods that should fill 70% of your plate (in no particular order). Obviously I cannot mention all the foods on the planet, but this will give you a good guide:

Good quality filtered water
Pumpkin seeds
Walnuts
Almonds
Chlorella
Spirulina

Himalayan salt
All grasses and green sea
    substances such as Wheat
    grass and Barley grass
Superfoods such as Maca
    and Bee pollen

Cucumbers are an incredible food and very alkaline, so never underestimate our juicy green friend. The same is true of:

Kale
Parsley
Spinach
Watercress
Rocket (basically anything
   green)
Sea vegetables
Sprouted foods
Soy beans
White haricot beans
Cayenne pepper
Garlic
Red pepper
Avocado
Beetroot
Broccoli
Cabbage
Celery
Collard/spring greens
Ginger
Green beans

Lettuce
Quinoa
Spelt
Goat's milk
Almond milk
Carrot
Horseradish
Swede
Turnip
Caraway seeds
Cumin seeds
Fennel seeds
Artichoke
Asparagus
Brussels sprouts
Cauliflower
Chives
Courgette
Leek
Peas
Rhubarb

Mustard greens
Okra
Onion
Radish
Sorrel
Tomato
Lentils
All herbs and spices
Coconut
Grapefruit
Lemon
Lime
Buckwheat
Avocado oil
Coconut oil
Evening primrose oil
Chia seeds
Sesame seed oil
Linseed oil
Olive oil
Udo's oil

Fruits that have a slightly higher sugar content (so eat less of these and always balance out with greens) which makes them not so alkalizing as our green vegetables but they still have fabulous health benefits:

Apple	Orange	Apricot
Pear	Papaya	Banana
Watermelon	Peach	Blackberry
Grapes	Pineapple	Blueberry
Guava	Raspberry	Cranberry
Honeydew melon	Strawberry	Fresh figs
Mango	Tangerine	Gooseberry

The following list contains mildly acidic foods (so keep your portions under control) but they have their health benefits so including them is good:

Black beans	Brazil nuts	Currants and dried fruits
Chickpeas	Hazelnuts	Fresh dates
Kidney beans	Pecans	Nectarine
Grape seed oil	Linseeds	Plum
Millet	Sunflower seeds	Sweet cherries

Highly acidic foods:

Beer	Yeast	Shellfish
Coffee	Pickled fruit	Veal
Lager	Corn	Cow's milk
Spirits	Oat bran	Cream
Wine	Rye	Cottage cheese
Carob	Beef	Hard cheese
Cocoa	Chicken	Ice cream
Jam	Eggs	Soy cheese
Malt mustard	Farm-raised fish	Yoghurt
Rice syrup	Organ meats	Cashews
Soy sauce	Pork	Peanuts
Vinegar	Poultry	Pistachios

White potatoes	Sugar (white or brown)	Maple syrup
Artificial sweeteners	Corn syrup	Molasses and all
Barley	Dried sugar cane	processed and packet
Malt	Fructose	foods
Syrup	Honey	

The other important thing to remember is to ensure your plate is full of the colours of the rainbow as the anti-inflammatory properties and health benefits are enormous.

When you look at the range of fresh fruits and vegetables available to us the colours are beautiful. Eating a rainbow diet in the form of fresh fruits and vegetables is the best thing you can do because each beautiful colour has its very own powerhouse of nutritional goodness. Each colour is caused by specific phytonutrients, which are natural chemicals that help protect the plants from germs, bugs, the sun's harmful rays and other potential threats that may stop it from thriving. The colours from the plant

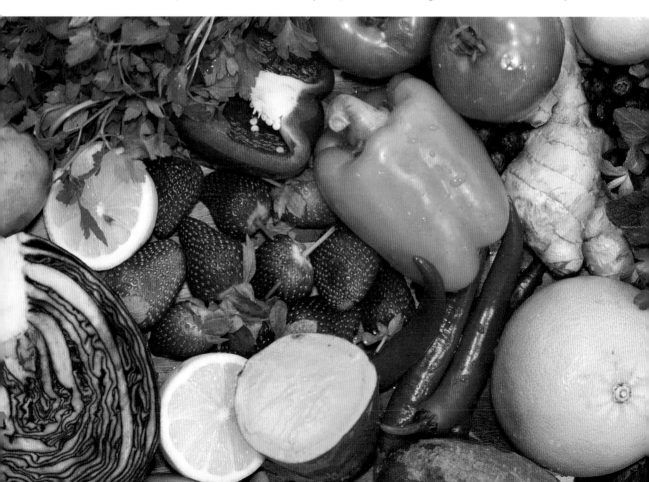

pigments have antioxidant properties and generally the more richly vibrant the colour the more antioxidants they contain. The ideal would be to include a little something from each colour at every meal. This way you can't go far wrong in your supply of vital vitamins and minerals. Not only this, but if you try adding each colour to every meal your plate will be pretty full, leaving very little room for junk or anything processed! Watch your skin change, your body tone up, and your brainpower expand in just a few short days. It's good to be reminded what health-giving qualities each and every fruit and vegetable can give you, because if you are dealing with an ailment right now, it will be a better guide to steer you in the right direction.

The rules are keep it simple and natural. Eating foods in their most natural state provides the maximum nutrients in an easily assimilated form. If you are sick, don't let it rule you. Flip it on its head and gain the energy you've always wanted. Take back control of your health, it could just be simpler than you think.

Top anti-inflammatory foods

Here is my A–Z of top anti-inflammatory foods for you to enjoy, and the reasons why:

Almonds: nuts are known for their anti-inflammatory properties, but some are better for you in this regard than others and almonds are right up there, with walnuts very close behind. They can specifically help with rheumatoid arthritis and are fabulous for the memory. They are a good alkalizing food and have been linked with muscle gain and helping to lower cholesterol. It's so easy to make your own almond milk too. Simply soak one cup of almonds (roughly 200g) in water for 8–12 hours or overnight. Rinse and peel off the skins and tip into a blender. Add four cups of water and blitz for several minutes until smooth. Then secure a muslin cloth over the bowl and pour the almond mixture through it. So easy and so nutritious!

Apples: they are abundant in fibre, and contain pectin, which has been shown to improve digestion. Pectin not only helps to stop diarrhoea-causing bacteria, it can add bulk to stools to enable them to pass easily through your system without drama. They also aid weight loss and reduce your risk of obesity. Apples are great for your teeth and, being nature's toothbrush due to their thick skin, can work like a scrubbing brush to reduce plaque and build-up to protect your teeth and stimulate your gums. Eating apples also produces saliva, providing a rinse to get rid of bacteria and food particles. A natural substance found in apples, called ursolic acid, can provide partial protection against fatty liver disease. In addition to the pectin they are also rich in malic acid that can aid the body in cleansing toxins, cholesterol, and carcinogens from your blood to promote a healthier liver. Apples can lower your risk of asthma, give you healthy bones, reduce your cancer risk, improve your eye health, strengthen your immune system, improve your brain power, and reduce your risk of heart attacks and stroke. So when the doctor said you should eat an apple a day, they were right!

Asparagus: delicious raw, this amazing anti-inflammatory superfood should be your go-to vegetable to use in meals as well as snacks. With its impressive anti-ageing properties, asparagus contains high amounts of vitamin A and C and is a great iron booster.

Avocado: I love avocados so much. They can be added to salads, smoothies, or just eaten as a snack. The healthy fats they contain make them a great choice for weight loss, reducing inflammation and supporting heart health, plus they are amazing for brain power and skin beauty. What's not to love?

Basil: herbs and spices are a great way to help reduce inflammation and when you add them to your food you are adding another level of health-enhancing goodness. Basil is considered a powerful anti-stress, anti-inflammatory, and immune-boosting agent. It contains an active ingredient called eugenol which has been linked to helping reduce the risk of cancer, heart disease, and diabetes, and has been shown to be as effective a painkiller as aspirin and ibuprofen. It's very alkalizing and extremely healing.

Beets: betalin is the powerful antioxidant that gives beet their robust colour and puts them high on the list of anti-inflammatory healing foods. Beets are rich in minerals such as potassium, magnesium, and calcium, and they boost nitric oxide production, greatly enhancing the circulation. Healing is proportionate to blood flow, so this is going to help speed things up.

Bell peppers: it's the flavonoids in bell peppers that give them their antioxidant and anti-inflammatory properties. It's also the reason why they're a superfood which can help enhance your health in many ways. You can use bell peppers for weight loss, as they are a low-calorie food, and the antioxidants they contain will help combat free radical damage within the body. Make sure you mix up the colours to get an all-round better fix.

Berries: blueberries and other antioxidant-laden berries like raspberries and blackberries are full of phytonutrients that give them their anti-inflammatory goodness. Antioxidants will not only contribute to protecting you from free radical damage and serious disease, but help to keep your memory tip-top as well.

Black beans: beans of all kinds are anti-inflammatory and are digested slowly by the body, making them great for weight loss. Because they contain a substantial amount of fibre they help to keep your body more regulated. They are loaded with antioxidants and protein, so are a great addition to your daily regime.

Broccoli: one of the top superfoods available, there really is almost nothing this vegetable can't do. It's high in fibre, and contains a loads of protein and phytochemicals, which are powerful antioxidants. It is a vitamin C powerhouse and has long been known to ward off certain diseases like cancer, but it's also helpful for many other illnesses and conditions too. It's easy to prepare, can be bought fresh or frozen, and used in many dishes or on its own. It's delicious when eaten raw and is an incredible anti-inflammatory food that should be included daily.

Buckwheat: contains catechins, tannins, rutin, and quercetin which are known to fight free radicals and inflammation. This is a popular food in Japan that will provide excellent anti-inflammatory results. It is great for replacing other foods that can lead to higher levels of inflammation such as white rice, white pastas, and white breads. Whole grains form an important part of an anti-inflammatory diet, and after fruits and vegetables are one of the staple foods you should be eating every day.

Cabbage: red cabbage should be your preferred choice so that you benefit from the anthocyanins it contains. These have been shown to provide a substantial anti-inflammatory benefit, but don't overlook other types of cabbage, as they are all part of the cruciferous family and will give an anti-inflammatory boost to any meal.

Cantaloupe: this contains phytonutrients that make it a powerful anti-inflammatory food and great for weight loss and with high levels of antioxidants. It also contains a ridiculous amount of vitamins A and C. Just be aware that it is a fruit and therefore does contain a higher amount of sugar, which is why you'll want to keep your portion sizes under control as it could be easy to overindulge.

Carrots: how can you not love carrots? I prefer them raw, like the majority of my vegetables, and snack on them throughout the day. They are crunchy and delicious and so nutritious, containing beta carotene, fibre, vitamin K, potassium, and antioxidants, making them the perfect protection against cancer, heart disease, eye problems, ageing skin, helping to prevent strokes and keep your teeth and gums healthy. Chop them, dip them, grate them, juice them … or just eat them!

Cauliflower: this is one of my favourite vegetables eaten raw. I don't enjoy it cooked, but love it raw with a nutritious dip as a snack during the day. Don't be fooled by its pale appearance: cauliflower contains the elusive vitamin K, and an impressive dose of vitamin C, as well as powerful antioxidants that alone make it worth eating. But it's the anti-inflammatory properties of cauliflower that make this white vegetable very deserving of a slot on your regular eating regime.

Celery: this is a powerful healing food and its antioxidants and anti-inflammatory properties have been shown to prevent heart disease and improve blood pressure, plus contributing to lower cholesterol. This little stick of goodness has a high potassium content which makes it great at flushing toxins out the body. Snack on it during the day to stop you reaching for the crisps and biscuits!

Cherries: these tasty little bundles can reduce blood pressure, help with inflammation, improve brain function, act as a great post-workout snack, and help you sleep. Cherries (particularly tart cherries) are a natural source of melatonin, the hormone that helps you control your sleep. Consuming a glass of cherry juice before you're off to bed can reduce the severity of insomnia and increase your overall sleep efficiency. Anyone affected by insomnia would do well to give this a go before reaching for the sleeping pills.

Coconut: the meaty, fleshy bit is considered a superfood because of its healing properties and its high levels of antioxidants. This highly nutritious, fibre-rich, multi-vitamin and mineral exotic food packs a mean punch when it comes to healthy foods.

Coriander: helps to reduce cholesterol, anaemia, and digestive problems. This wonderful health-giving herb is rich in calcium, iron, and vitamin C. Sprinkle on all your salads or pop into your smoothie for extra goodness.

Cucumber: I love them, I add them to my juice every morning, chop them for the children daily, and quite frankly should run my own farm or have shares in them, because in my household we literally eat tons of them. Cucumbers are the fourth most cultivated vegetable in the world and known to be one of the best foods for your body's overall health, often referred to as a superfood. Cucumbers can be sprayed with pesticides, so it is important to buy organic or even better, grow them yourself. If you can't buy organic, peel them before eating. They are a great 'pick me up' as they are a fantastic source of B vitamins. They boost your vitamin intake and also rehydrate the body because they are 95% water, helping to eliminate toxins. Cucumber can be used brilliantly for skin irritations and sunburn. If you place a slice over puffy eyes, its anti-inflammatory properties help reduce swelling, and the silicon and sulphur in cucumbers is said to stimulate hair growth. Cucumbers contribute to warding off several types of cancer, including breast, ovarian, uterine, and prostate.

For bad breath, you can take a slice of cucumber and press it to the roof of your mouth with your tongue for 30 seconds and the phytochemicals will kill the bacteria in your mouth. Cucumbers also contain enough sugar, B vitamins, and electrolytes to replenish many essential nutrients, reducing the intensity of both hangovers and headaches. This juicy vegetable can also relieve constipation, reduce cholesterol, and control blood pressure. The juice contains a hormone needed by the cells of the pancreas for producing insulin, which has been found to be beneficial to diabetic patients. Cucumber is an excellent source of silica, which is known to help promote joint health by strengthening the connective tissues and is a rich source of vitamins A, B1, B6, C, and D; folate; calcium; magnesium; and potassium. When mixed with carrot juice, they can relieve gout and arthritic pain by lowering uric acid levels. Eat them, juice them, and snack on them as often as you can!

Dark chocolate: while you'll want to go easy with it, you are still able to enjoy dark chocolate as a sweet treat that is also somewhat anti-inflammatory. Try to avoid milk chocolate, as this actually falls on the inflammatory side of the equation. Milk chocolate is generally mixed with hefty amounts of processed sugar and doesn't contain the same antioxidants and other properties that make dark chocolate OK as a little sweet treat from time to time.

Fennel: the health benefits of fennel have been known for quite some time now, but the more that's discovered about it, the more it shows up on lists of healthy foods. It ranks high on my anti-inflammatory list due to its strong phytonutrient and antioxidant count, which together help treat the symptoms, as well as the cause, of inflammation in the body. It also adds great flavour to any meal.

Flaxseed: the lignans and alpha-linolenic acids in flaxseed help provide a big surge of anti-inflammatory goodness and it's as easy as sprinkling some seeds into a soup or smoothie. The omega 3 content is such a big part of eating an anti-inflammatory diet that it's a daily must-have!

Garlic: garlic is one anti-inflammatory food that most of us can agree on as definitely having the ability to battle inflammation and boost your immune system. Garlic supplements are often prescribed as a way to help with chronic inflammation, but an easier way is to simply start using more of it in your meals. If anyone I know has a fever or cold/flu I tell them to crush it on a spoon and glug it down with some water. I'm not going to lie, it's horrible, but the viruses or bacteria literally go away! They may hate me temporarily, and stink a little bit, but then I hear them recommending it to other people!

Ginger: containing a fabulous amount of antioxidants, ginger is a very cleansing root, so you'll find this in detox teas and recipes, as it also helps to clear out the digestive system. It can relieve nausea, motion sickness, pain, and inflammation and is a fabulous addition to smoothies, juices, and soups. You can grate it, chew on it, add to all your drinks, and generally feast on this wonderful food daily!

Grapefruit: while the red/pink grapefruit has a higher nutritional content, the yellow one is not flagging too far behind. This slightly sharper tasting fruit still contains an amazing amount of vitamin C, ranking third behind oranges and lemons. It helps the body to metabolize protein properly and has been used by many people as a weight loss aid over the years. Half a grapefruit before meals may start to fill you up, so you eat fewer calories, plus it can also improve skin appearance and tone.

Kale: kale is an absolute must-have when it comes to nutrient-dense, alkaline living. It has to be one of the most abundant sources of nutrients on earth, delicious, dark green (so full of chlorophyll), and hugely alkaline. To super-nourish, re-energize, revitalize, and thrive I really suggest you have this as often as possible. Kale boasts huge amounts of vitamins A, C, and K, as well as sulphur-containing phytonutrients. Kale is one of the most antioxidant-rich foods we can consume and the preventative benefits of kale are linked to the combination of the strong antioxidants called carotenoids and flavonoids. It contains significant levels of at least 45 different antioxidants, all of which play a role in fighting against conditions linked to oxidative stress and inflammation. And remember, oxidative stress is another name for the body breaking down and ageing quickly. So if you want to feel good, look good, and be nourished inside and out, kale is the way to go. One of the greatest benefits of kale is its anti-inflammatory effect due to its omega 3 and huge vitamin K content. It can help protect against bladder, breast, colon, ovarian, and prostate cancers. When we eat kale, fibre-related nutrients bind with certain bile acids in the intestine and pass out of the body. When this happens the liver has to replace these bile acids and draws upon our existing cholesterol supply, which lowers our cholesterol. Kale is also rich in eye-health-promoting lutein and zeaxanthin compounds which can help prevent macular degeneration. Kale is full of fibre, making it fantastic for the digestive system, and it contains glucosinolates, which means it helps protect our stomach lining from bacterial overgrowth (of bad bacteria such as Helicobacter pylori). Last but not least, kale assists in detoxifying the body by collecting toxins such as heavy metals, pesticides, and herbicides and then taking them straight out of the body!

Lemons and limes: if there is one thing my fruit bowl is never allowed to run out of in my house its lemons and limes. Not only do I love them and add to all my water, squeeze them on my avocados and just about any other dish I can, I like the look and smell of having them in my kitchen. They have so many mind-blowing qualities it's hard not to love them. Firstly, they act as a digestive and detoxifying aid. If you squeeze some juice onto your hands, you will see how soft they make your skin feel. Imagine what a beautiful effect that lemon is going to have on your liver. Secondly, drinking juice with lemon/lime in every morning helps to stabilize your body's pH balance (in its natural state lemon is acidic, but once ingested it becomes alkalizing) and gives you the best immune boost due to its high vitamin C content. Lemons and limes also contribute to reducing your risk of cancers, protect you against anaemia, help prevent kidney stones, and support your heart health. You can use the juice in your hair, on your skin, to fragrance the room, to clean the work surfaces. There's no end to their talents!

Lentils: these are a great addition to any diet because they're a slow carbohydrate that doesn't spike your blood sugar levels, they contain fibre to help keep you regular, and protein to help you meet your daily needs. They are an anti-inflammatory food and are easy to use because they cook up comparatively quickly. You can use them as a side or main dish or in soups, adding texture and thickness as well as healthy properties.

Mangoes: if you want flawless skin, here's your answer! Mangoes cleanse your skin from deep inside by helping treat pores and giving you an array of vitamins and minerals at the same time. It is known as the love fruit, as it has aphrodisiac qualities, especially improving virility in you guys! It's said that mangoes increase love and passion, and give you white, healthy eyes as they are loaded with vitamin A. Also, if you have digestive complaints this could be the natural medicine that you have been looking for. It has a high enzyme content, so helps break down protein, and being loaded with fibre helps aid fabulous digestion. On a hot summer's day this fruit can physically help to cool you down. They are high in antioxidants, particularly helping protect the body against leukaemia and breast cancer, and cancer, prostate cancer. The leaves of the mango are excellent for diabetes. Simply boil five or six mango leaves in a pan and the liquor can help to regulate diabetes. Being so rich in vitamin C and A and a variety of carotenoids, these nutrients will keep your immune system particularly happy.

Millet: a grain that does not contain gluten, and a very easy alternative to wheat. It's a natural supplier of iron, protein, and calcium and keeps your body more on the alkalizing side of life!

Mint: add to water, salads, or use as a tea. This mint provides great flavour and is easily grown at home. It provides vitamins and minerals and has a ton of alkalizing properties.

Mung beans: linked to lowering cholesterol, fighting certain types of cancer, and supporting diabetes, mung beans contribute to strengthening the immune system and provide iron, fibre, antioxidants, and a raft of nutrients that are beneficial to the whole body, including your digestive system.

Oats: go for the basic variety of oats and opt out of the instant oatmeal with added flavours and sugars that you find on supermarket shelves. This anti-inflammatory food will give you an abundance of energy and you can add your own fruit and nuts to this, too. Oats consistently rank as one of the healthier foods you can eat, specifically as a way to keep your heart healthy and maintain a proper weight. A breakfast of oatmeal is one way to stabilize blood sugars and provide yourself with sustainable energy and no crash.

Oranges: we are all aware of their high vitamin C content and their ability to ward off colds, but that's not all these delicious juicy fruits can do. They are an unbelievable source of fibre, which keeps the intestines and bowel happy, as well as supplying good amounts of vitamins A and B. They also contain calcium and potassium, so help to keep your bones and electrolytes in tip-top shape. Although on the more acidic side and with the high sugar level of fruit, their health benefits are massive. Just one orange a day (alongside your other rainbow choices) can help protect against heart disease and cancer and provide anti-inflammatory and antiviral properties.

Papaya: its main pain-reducing ingredient is proteolytic enzyme papain, which can be just as effective as non-steroidal anti-inflammatory drugs. Papaya is not a top-selling fruit, but it is one of the healthiest anti-inflammatory fruits you can eat. That's because there are ingredients in papaya that aren't found in other fruits, which particularly gives it the edge on inflammation. It's high in antioxidants and beta carotene and helps massively at improving the digestion.

Parsley: an excellent source of vitamin C, which assists in reducing free radicals, parsley provides you with one of the most important B vitamins, folic acid, and calcium.

Peas: a decent underestimated food for high mineral content and vitamins. They have been shown to reduce the chances of heart disease and stroke due to their ability to prevent damage to cells. They are anti-ageing and healthy for the environment because peas work with bacteria in the soil to fix nitrogen from the air and deposit it in the soil. This reduces the need for artificial fertilizers since one of their main ingredients is nitrogen. They give is healthy bones, reduce cholesterol, and prevent constipation.

Pineapple: rich in digestive enzymes, this luscious and delicious anti-inflammatory fruit can reduce swelling, bruising, musculoskeletal injuries, arthritis, and tendinitis and can help relieve digestive complaints as well as cleaning up damaged cells. You can enjoy it any way you like, either by preparing it fresh, or using frozen in smoothies for your morning energy boost! Those that are watching their blood sugar levels to prevent or manage diabetes should check to see how their bodies handle it and keep portion sizes to suit.

Quinoa: it has a fantastic amount of both protein and fibre, and an eclectic mix of vitamins and minerals so your body gets exactly what it needs. Mix it with your salads and cover with delicious dressings to give you more filling substance to your food.

Red onions: eating just one to two onions a day has been associated with the greatest benefit in reducing colorectal, oral, laryngeal, oesophageal, and ovarian cancers. Red onions are super-rich in quercetin, so eat them in their natural form rather than via supplementation. They can help with a whole list of ailments that they help such as easing stiffness and swelling from arthritis, lowering your risk of cancers and inhibiting tumour growth, preventing heart disease, reducing severity of bladder infections, and helps to prevent allergies, coughs, and earaches. They are rich in chromium which lowers blood sugar and boosts your sex drive, relieves stomach aches and gives you radiant glowing skin. I know they are not the most sociable of foods, so if you are worried about 'onion breath' especially when consuming the onion raw (which is the best) just make sure you eat plenty of green veggies, such as dandelions, parsley or coriander for fresh breath. Or try chewing on rosemary, fennel or peppermint as an alternative.

Rocket: is a great detox green leafy vegetable and contains a good deal of goodness, providing 16% of your daily calcium requirements, 47% of your vitamin A, and 8% of your iron per 100 grams. It helps protect against cancer, contributes to maintaining a

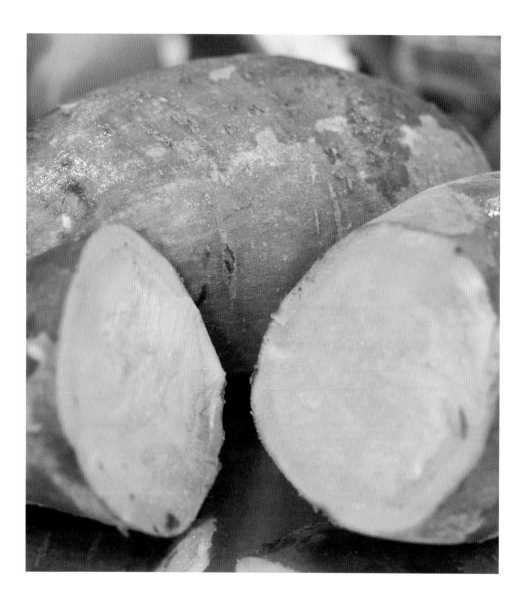

healthy heart, is good for your bones, and great for the complexion. Add to your salads or smoothies for added vigour!

Shiitake mushrooms: for a long time we've known about the benefits of shiitake mushrooms to the immune system, but it's only been recently recognized as an anti-inflammatory food because these mushrooms contain specific substances called poly-saccharides that provide the anti-inflammatory benefits we need.

Spinach: this green leaf is something we should all eat more of since it is one of the most nutrient-dense vegetables available to us. It is full of fibre, phytonutrients, and protein, and an incredible anti-inflammatory food if you wish to avoid things like heart disease and cancer. It's a great choice to mix with your fruits in your daily smoothie and can be easily added to salads, wraps, and soups for alkalizing goodness.

Sweet potatoes: this inexpensive vegetable is very underestimated. To start with, I bet you wouldn't think that they are an excellent source of vitamin D? If you have thyroid issues then these are your babies! Sweet potatoes are also amazing for your teeth, bones, skin, and nervous system. They help improve constipation, because of the high fibre content, and their ability to clean the digestive tract and reduce the possibility of stomach ulcers, particularly when the sweet potato is juiced raw is incredible. Sweet potatoes are an amazing source of magnesium, which is great if you are stressed and exhausted since magnesium helps relax both the muscles and the mind. They contain good amounts of iron, increasing your white cell formation, which helps to ward off disease and viruses. They also aid in stopping muscle cramps, provide you with high levels of vitamin C, and if you are trying for a baby, they are high in folate, which also supports foetal development. Juice them, grate them, eat them raw, or bake them, boil them, mash them, and eat them! In my opinion raw is best, but just find some way of getting them into your daily regime.

Tomatoes: these red beauties are loaded to the max with great health benefits. They are incredible for skin beauty, both when eaten and when applied topically to the skin. When it comes to prostate, colorectal, and stomach cancers, they offer one of the best forms of antioxidant protection because of their lycopene content. They have high amounts of calcium and vitamin K, making them excellent for maintaining strong bones, not only for maintenance, but when repairing fractures. They contain coumaric acid and chlorogenic acid which work to protect the body from carcinogens produced from cigarette smoke. So, if you have been a puffer in your time, include a few of these in your daily regime and you could just help to turn back time. Tomatoes also contain B vitamins and potassium in abundance so they can lower blood pressure, prevent heart attacks and strokes, and protect you from other life-threatening diseases.

Turnips: they contain high amounts of vitamin K and their omega 3s make them a surprising source of this essential fat. They also pack a punch in the vitamin C department.

Watercress: one way of adding zing to your lettuce leaves is to add some watercress, not only to enhance the flavour of your salads, but also to truly boost the nutritional value on your plate. Watercress is absolutely bursting with vitamins and minerals. It is fast growing and one of the oldest known leaf vegetables consumed by human beings. It has also been known to help normalize blood pressure and cholesterol levels within the body, which as we all know are major problems. It can increase our sex drive and enhance fertility and breast milk production, so it is fantastic in more ways than one! Plus, not only does it greatly improve mental function, it also helps with our memory and abilities to concentrate and absorb new information. This wonderful little green superfood may also aid prevention of certain cancers such as breast, colon, prostate, and lung, and it also contains lutein, which helps prevent artery and cell damage. It is very low in calories, high in potassium, and acts as a diuretic drawing excess fluid down and out of the body, helping remove toxins and acidic waste. It regulates the flow of bile, aids digestion, and relieves bleeding gums. It improves the complexion, strengthens bones and teeth and is a fantastic folk remedy for treating allergies, watery eyes, sneezing and stuffy heads. And if that wasn't enough to convince you, due to its high iodine content, it has a fantastic strengthening effect on the thyroid gland.

Watermelon: this has to be one of my all-time favourite fruits. I love it in salads, in my morning juice, and just on its own for a snack. Watermelon is a great source of lycopene which may help decrease the risk of heart disease by lowering LDL cholesterol. And it reduces the risk for certain cancers, primarily prostate, as well as the risk of macular degeneration. It improves blood vessel function and lowers stroke risk. It's also rich in a phytonutrient called citrulline which can work well as a treatment for mild to moderate erectile dysfunction. Watermelons are a great source of hydration and energy and have been known to reduce the severity of asthma attacks and support weight loss. They can also help protect nerve function by eradicating inflammation. Watermelons help your delicate pH balance due to the high potassium levels and can be an important support when it comes to your digestive health because of the high fibre and high water content.

Winter squash: a seriously nutritionally power-packed vegetable, being high in vitamins A, B6, C, folate, magnesium, fibre, riboflavin, phosphorus, potassium, and manganese, this vegetable will help you process fats and carbohydrates; help prevent high blood pressure, strokes, and heart disease; reduce inflammation; and promote good digestion. Add it to your soups and stews and you have yourself a healthy meal.

Recommendation: swapping one of your unhealthy treats for two anti-inflammatory foods each day will make such a difference to how you feel! Small change. Big results!

CHAPTER 12

MY TOP 12 HERBS AND SPICES

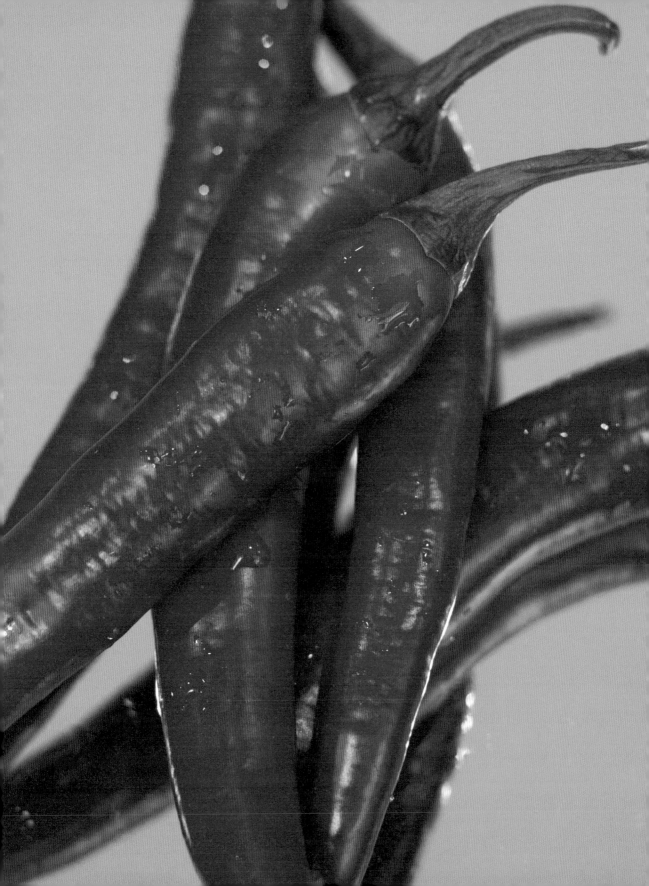

Your extra health insurance. Use herbs as your medicine … because your body will love you for it!

Herbs are superfoods and should be included as much as possible in your diet as they offer a vast amount of nourishment to the body and are a subject all on their own. But I wanted to include some common, easy to use varieties for you so that you can always be in tip-top condition and create fabulous health always. You will notice some of these are in the anti-inflammatory and alkalizing lists, but you can be confident in the knowledge that all herbs are good for you in one way or another. You can use them to correct acute and chronic conditions, but just understanding their purpose helps you to choose which ones you need, and adding these as much as possible into your daily regime will help to protect you on a whole new level.

Aloe vera: this has been listed as a superfood as it contains 75 healing compounds, including natural steroids, antibiotic agents, amino acids, minerals, and enzymes. It has been used since Egyptian times as a beauty skin moisturizer and heals burns, cuts, bruises, acne, and eczema. Also, taken internally aloe alkalizes the digestive track preventing over-acidity, which is the most common cause of digestive complaints such as acid reflux, heartburn, and ulcers. We always have a large plant growing somewhere in our house and just pick a leaf or two off to use on the skin. If you burn yourself it's like a small miracle. I scalded my head on my hair straighteners recently and the skin on my temple was really red and tight. It was so sore. Within 30 seconds of putting the aloe gel on the burn it had completely disappeared as if it had never happened. It's in the gel that all the goodness is stored, the vitamins, minerals, amino acids, and antioxidants.

Black pepper: the piperine in black pepper is a powerful cancer-fighting ingredient and becomes twice as potent when combined with turmeric. The spice has an array of antioxidants that help remove harmful free radicals, protecting the body from cancers and other diseases. It also contains vitamin C, vitamin A, and flavonoids. To derive the greatest goodness from black pepper eat it freshly ground and do not cook it too much. Black pepper helps to stimulate the digestion by encouraging the secretion of hydrochloric acid, which in turn helps digest protein, and it stimulates the enzyme activity in your liver which helps to keep the cleansing process of the liver working efficiently. It also contributes to the stimulation of the brain, making it more active, and improves the skin by increasing blood circulation (you can also use it topically by adding it to honey as an exfoliator). It's also very effective if you suffer from vitiligo, where the skin loses pigmentation and creates white patches. Due to its antibacterial content, a teaspoon of honey with freshly crushed pepper helps relieve colds, coughs, and chest congestion.

Chilli peppers: containing capsaicin, love them or hate them, you know these little spicy friends can benefit you in many ways. For starters they can help improve migraines by desensitizing and lessening the original pain as the body gets distracted due to the hot sensation! That is a real theory and one which has been known to work. It also relieves joint pain in a similar fashion. It can be applied to the skin to reduce pain: the pain receptors exhaust themselves and deplete the body's reserves. Once this happens the capsaicin acts as a pain reliever, and can be used effectively, too, with shingles, HIV, and neuropathy. Chilli peppers can help reduce skin conditions such as psoriasis, and fight flu, colds, and fungal infections, as they are full of beta carotene and anti-oxidants that help support your immune system. Nasal sprays that contain capsaicin are amazing at reducing congestion, so no medication is needed. They combat bad breath, help with allergies and irritation, and promote weight loss by revving up your metabolic rate.

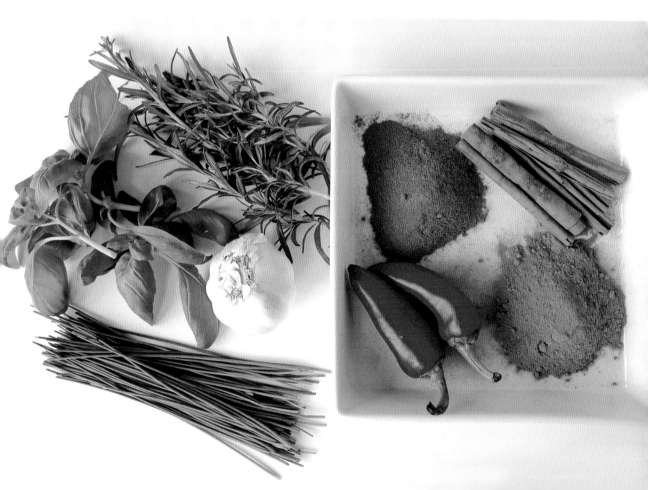

Capsaicin is also known for reducing the growth of cancer cells due to its massively powerful anti-inflammatory properties. So try adding some to your foods on a regular basis.

Cinnamon: This spice has such powerful medicinal properties and you can add it to almost everything. If you look at the history of cinnamon it dates back as far as the ancient Egyptians and was regarded as rare and valuable and fit for kings. Well, they were not far wrong. It's loaded with antioxidant and anti-inflammatory properties. It has been linked to a reduction in the risk of cardiovascular disease, and as little as 1 gram per day has been shown to reduce diabetes. It lowers cholesterol, and reduces the growth of cancer cells as it is a potent activator of detoxifying enzymes in the colon, protecting against further cancerous growths. It has incredible antibacterial and antifungal properties and is especially helpful when it comes to its respiratory properties. Trials are also taking place to test how effective cinnamon is against HIV infection, which shows just how amazing this herb is when it comes to boosting your immune system. It's delicious, protects your health, and gives your body the medicine that it needs.

Cloves: much more healing than you might think and so much more than just a seasoning for your food. They contain important nutrients and are high in antioxidants. They include an ingredient called eugenol, which helps to stop oxidative damage caused by toxins and other chemicals. Ground cloves are high in vitamin C and this can provide support to your immune system. Clove oil has been strongly linked to aiding in protection against oesophageal cancer cells. Cloves can kill off bacteria including E. coli that are linked to diarrhoea and fatigue and can be highly effective when it comes to oral health. It is said to improve your liver function and reverse signs of cirrhosis and scarring of the liver. Some compounds in cloves have been shown to preserve bone mass making it great for osteoporosis. Cloves are also useful in preventing stomach ulcers as they increase the production of gastric mucus. They can also help keep your blood sugar levels in check as they contain nigericin which is found to increase the uptake of sugar from the blood into cells and improve the function of cells that produce insulin.

Coriander: acting like a little Pacman, helping to remove toxins from the body, this wonderful herb is also a powerful antioxidant. It helps scavenge free radicals and fights against cell migration. Helping to prevent cancer it also balances blood sugar levels, making it extremely helpful for diabetes. It can aid in lowering cholesterol, making it a great food source for heart health. Coriander also has potent antifungal and antimicrobial effects and can break down the cell wall of pathogens, preventing them from proliferating. With more research needed, it is thought, at this stage, that coriander is showing massive potential for helping prevent the progression of diseases such as Alzheimer's and other forms of dementia, as it can help promote good memory. The leaves, stems, roots, and seeds of the whole plant can be used, or for an even more potent form, you can purchase coriander oil and add a few drops to water or juice, or pop it straight under your tongue.

Ginger: I love ginger and try to use it most days in my juices, smoothies, or soups. It is right up there with the other super herbs such as turmeric and contains the compound gingerol, a natural anti-inflammatory and antioxidant. It can curb an overactive immune system and support the body in many ways. It can treat many forms of nausea, especially morning sickness, gas, irritable bowel and diarrhoea and has been shown to be helpful for cancer patients when suffering side effects from chemotherapy. It's amazing at reducing muscle pain and soreness and the anti-inflammatory effects can help with osteoarthritis. It also helps protect the heart and lowers cholesterol levels and its gingerol component may protect you against cancer too. It is a powerful protector against age-related cognitive decline, and lowers your risk of infection as it inhibits the growth of many different types of bacteria.

Ginseng: the ultimate herb for handling stress. This is widely known as an energizing tonic and is particularly beneficial when recovering from an illness or surgery for its restorative and anti-infective properties. It promotes regeneration from stress and fatigue, lowers blood sugar and cholesterol levels, promotes relaxation, treats diabetes, and helps to manage sexual dysfunction in men. You want ginseng that contains natural ginsenosides and I prefer the powdered type as you can control exactly the amount that you take. I would suggest no more than 1–2 teaspoons per day, which you can add to your green smoothie or take off the spoon.

Nettle: yes, the type that grows in your garden and is classed as a weed. You can juice it, make it into a tea, but just be careful when you pick it! It might sting so you may need to wear gloves. Nettles are a great immune booster and incredible body cleanser. They contain antioxidants that help defend your cells against free radical damage and protect you from serious disease. A cup of nettle tea in the morning is an ideal way to get your bowels moving and release mucus in the colon allowing for better flushing of excess waste. Nettle offers an array of minerals and vitamins and is great to increase thyroid function. It also helps flush the kidneys and bladder to prevent and soothe urinary tract infections. These little leaves will also reduce inflammation, relieve allergies, help muscle and joint pain, strengthen your heart, and boost your immune system.

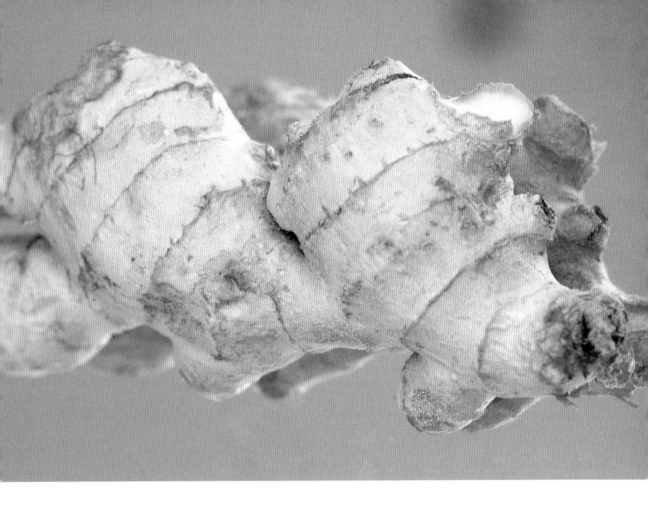

Parsley: this tasty green leaf is so much more than a natural breath freshener and has a surprising amount of healing abilities. Did you know that half a cup of fresh parsley contains 40 milligrams of vitamin C? That's more than half the amount found in a whole orange. It's also incredibly healing, thanks to its two main components. It contains myristicin and apiol, both of which can help increase the flow of urine. Passing more urine helps remove infection-causing bacteria from the urinary tract. It is this same diuretic action that also helps prevent premenstrual bloating. Nibbling away on parsley for a few days before menstruation can help increase urine flow, removing excess fluids from the body before the discomfort begins.

Parsley is a great source of folate, a B vitamin that is necessary for producing red blood cells and helping to prevent birth defects. It also contains large amounts of vitamins A, C, K, and iron. The myristicin, an organic compound found in the essential oil of parsley, not only inhibits tumour formation (especially in the lungs), but also activates the enzymes, which helps to fight against oxidized molecules and free radicals in the body. Myristicin can also neutralize carcinogens (toxins) like benzopyrene in cigarette

smoke that can pass through the body, consequently fighting against colon and prostate cancer. Parsley is rich with an antioxidant arsenal that includes luteolin, a flavonoid
that searches out and eradicates free radicals in the body that cause oxidative stress in
cells and acts as an anti-inflammatory agent. When consumed regularly, parsley is a
powerful herb to help fight against osteoarthritis and rheumatoid arthritis. Being high
in vitamin A helps the important lymphocytes, or white blood cells, to fight infection
in the body. Helping to prevent heart disease and support our nervous system, I think
it's fair to say we should not underestimate this common herb. Next time you are using
parsley as just a garnish, think about adding a little more to your plate on a daily basis.
It's the small changes that make the biggest differences!

Rosemary: this wonder herb grows wild in many parts of the world, especially in warm
and sunny climates. Used in aromatherapy oils it can help with concentration, making
it a fantastic choice if you are sitting an exam or test of some type. It also helps lower
stress levels, particularly when combined with lavender oil and has been said to improve
mental energy where there is a need to be inspired and have fresh mental clarity. It has
been linked to hair growth, particularly in conditions like alopecia, and when rubbed on
the scalp has shown signs of improvement due to its stimulatory effects. When eaten
it is a rich source of iron, calcium, and B vitamins, and is well known for helping with
muscle aches and pains and boosting the immune and circulatory systems.

Turmeric: if you have pain and disease or discomfort in your body then look no
further. Curcumin is the main ingredient in this incredible spice and it has massively
powerful anti-inflammatory effects as well as being an extremely strong antioxidant. If
you want to experience the full effects of this spice you need large doses, so it would
be advisable to take a supplement that contains high amounts of curcumin, and if you
are adding lashings of this into your food remember to add black pepper too as it will
help your body to absorb better into your blood stream. This orange power powder
also helps to support your brain, lowering your risk of heart disease as it improves the
function of the endothelium, which is the lining of your blood vessels. It helps regulate
blood pressure and blood clotting. It has been a contributor to the death of cancer
cells and reduces the growth of new blood vessels in tumours. Many of my arthritic
clients have benefited so much from curcumin supplements as it improves aches and
pains massively. It's also fantastic for treating depression as it boosts brain-derived neu-
rotrophic factors, potentially reversing a shrinking hippocampus, the area of the brain
which has a role in memory and learning. It is also said to boost serotonin and dopamine, the two main chemicals which raise mood.

CHAPTER 13

EXTRA TOOLS IN YOUR TOOLBOX

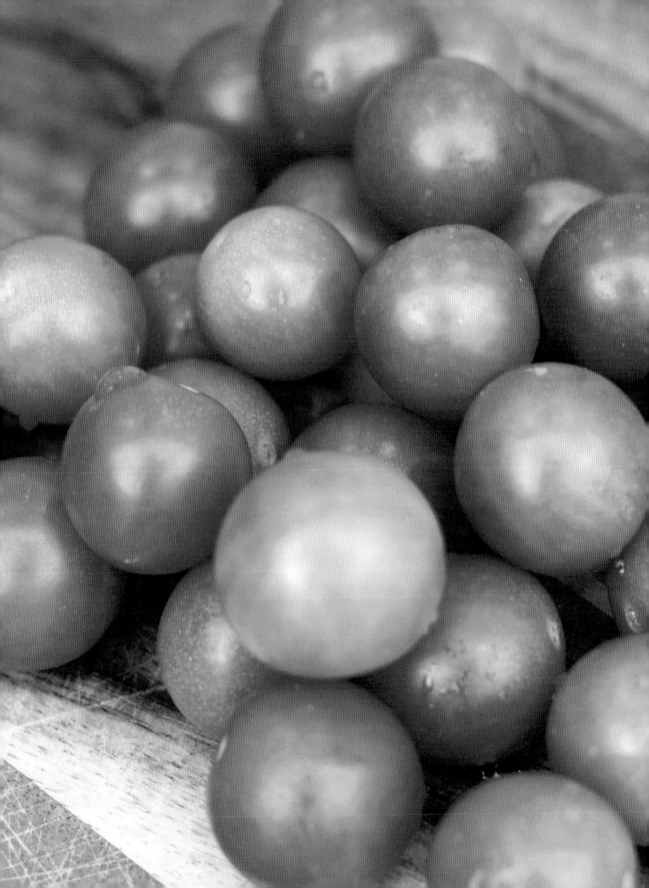

In the world of health, there are so many things to talk about that it's hard to know where to draw the line. Ultimately, I think all we want is to feel utterly fabulous each and every day and have as much energy as possible in order to maintain brain power, to build our new business, have a ton of babies, fly helicopters, meet new friends, sail round the world, run a marathon, meet the Queen, fall in love, plant a herb garden, climb a mountain, do a skydive, learn how to cook, perform on stage, learn a new language, change jobs, go scuba diving, attend a music festival! Whatever your wants and wishes, the art of giving your body what it needs to stay in the best shape possible is one that you can and will develop over time. So here are a few extra things you can have up your sleeve to help you in your journey getting there.

Sprouting seeds

Adding sprouted seeds into your diet could be one of the most health-enhancing additions you can make. They are 100% natural and pure and one of the most healthful, economical, life-force energy foods you can have. The key to successful sprouting is making sure you rinse and drain well, and that way you will never be without the perfect sprouts to sprinkle on your food, eat as a snack, or add to your smoothies. Investing in some proper sprouting jars is highly advisable. This is a really good investment for the years of use you can obtain from them. You only need two jars and can continuously produce amazing superfoods with this method.

Sprouting is an alternative word for germinating but sprouting goes beyond that and results in a partially grown young plant. You can sprout anything from nuts, seeds (such as radish, kale, broccoli, etc), beans, pulses, legumes, or grains. The benefit of sprouting is that it provides enhanced amino acids, vitamins, and minerals for your body in a very natural way. When a seed is soaked, the plant's enzyme inhibitors are removed and a whole chain of reactions begins. As the plant grows at a rapid rate, the vitamin content increases dramatically, to the point where the sprouted seed can contain hundreds and thousands of times more nourishment than it did previously. Then the protein, carbohydrates, and fats begin to break down into a predigested form. The enzymes of each seed, bean, nut, or grain also skyrocket, making sprouts one of the richest enzyme foods on the planet.

They can help with many ailments, such as digestive issues and immunity problems, boosting your circulation, and improving your heart health, your eyesight, your bone, skin, and muscle strength, and halting premature ageing. The best and most health-enhancing sprouts to begin with are: broccoli seeds, radish seeds, mung beans, lentils, fenugreek, chickpeas, and quinoa. As an example of their enormous goodness, a three-day old broccoli sprout contains between 20 and 100 times more goodness than the broccoli itself. That's not to say you should stop eating broccoli, but having the sprouted seeds too is going to give you such a nutritional hit of amazingness, it would be crazy not to. Sprouted seeds contain chemicals that disarm free radicals, preventing harmful diseases, and give the body the fighting materials that it needs to stay energetic and well.

It's really easy to do if you follow these simple rules. Make sure the jar that you choose is clean and oil free. Use just a small handful of one type of seeds (because they expand in the jar). Pour clean water onto your seeds, up to an inch over the level of the seeds. Then cover the jar (if it's not a professional sprouting jar) with a mesh lid. All that matters here is that nothing else can get into the jar except air. And that is a must! Leave the jar with the water in to soak overnight.

The next morning, drain off the water thoroughly and rinse the contents of your jar. Drain off the water by preferably leaving the jar upside down. This is the point at which your sprouting could potentially go wrong. If you do not drain properly and leave them in water your seeds could go rancid before they sprout (you would smell it if this happens). You must drain and leave them without water. You then need to rinse your sprouts twice a day, draining each time. Leave them in the light, but not in direct sunlight. Within two to five days your little seeds will be showing baby shoots, and this is when they are ready to eat. Then you can pop them in an airtight container and keep them in the fridge. They will last for at least five days! You can then begin sprouting

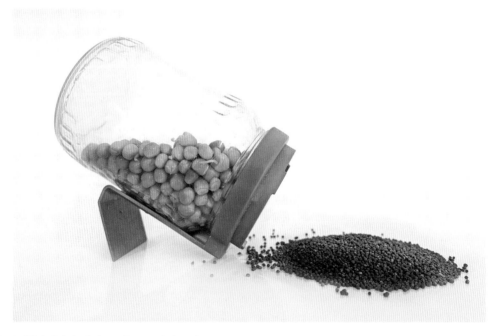

your next new jar so you always have an array of fresh sprouts on the go and can add them to everything you eat!

Dry skin brushing

This is great for the appearance of your skin as well as detoxing. One of the best ways I know to help you get fabulous-looking skin on your legs, bum, tum, and arms is skin brushing. This technique can be used whether you are male or female and it is not just about vanity. Your skin is an important route of elimination, and on an average day can get rid of at least 10% of your metabolic waste. That's why the Chinese call it the third lung. The lymphatic system does not have a pump in the way the blood has the heart, so skin brushing helps to stimulate the lymphatic system to enable toxins to be removed from the body. After all, it is the build-up of toxins and acids within the body that create disease, so it is vital to keep everything flowing within the body to remain healthy. Life is constantly moving and that is how our bodies should function, too. Never standing still or stagnating. Skin brushing removes dead skin cells on the surface allowing the skin to breathe and also improves the texture and appearance, giving you a firmer and more glowing look and feel. Skin is extremely absorbent, like a large sponge, and care also needs to be taken when using anti-perspirants, as they can clog up the lymph under the arm and allow the introduction of heavy metals like aluminum into the body.

Skin brushing is a great way of making changes to give you better health if you do it daily. You will need a non-synthetic bristle that can be found in most good health stores. It is helpful to choose one with a long detachable handle so you can reach your back. Start on the soles of the feet, and then brush in small strokes up the feet, ankles, calves, thighs, and buttocks. Then brush up the front and back of the torso as far as the heart. Work up the hands and arms and then down the neck, chest and upper back to the heart. Avoid brushing the face, as the skin is too sensitive and only brush gently over the breast area.

Hot and cold showers

Combining both hot and cold water when you shower has amazing therapeutic benefits for your body. When cold water hits the body it causes the blood to move closer to the inner organs to keep them warm. This increases the overall blood circulation in your body. The cold water also helps to reduce stress by numbing the nervous system and rejuvenating the skin. It boosts the immune system and leaves you feeling more energetic because cold water increases your oxygen intake and heart rate, leaving you feeling ready for the day! The hot part of your shower can help to reduce tension in your muscles and is a great stress reliever. It can help relieve congestion and can also improve blood flow by expanding blood vessels. This is a great combination and can work wonders for your energy levels. I would suggest one minute each of hot and cold for 10 minutes per day.

Make your mealtimes sacred

It's easy to have mealtimes turn into a business, quick to eat so that we can move on to the next activity. Perhaps in the chaos you've lost family mealtimes all together? There are real benefits to sitting down and enjoying a meal with the people you love. Mealtimes should be a candlelit, sacred celebration of the day's events, a time for sharing stories, dreams, and a time to grow as a family, or as a couple, or simply time to 'be' and reflect on your day. When you cook with love and eat with attention, you are taking in the very stuff of life. Also showing gratitude before each meal and blessing your food before you eat can give you a deeper level of appreciation. Some people have very little food, so when we have it in abundance it is certainly something to be thankful for.

Fasting and healing

Don't panic, I'm not about to give you a religious education lesson, but I just wanted to point out a few connections between fasting and the way we feel about food and health, mentally and physically. Fasting has been carried out for centuries and is now considered one of the best and fastest ways to heal the body from disease and ailments. It is without doubt one of the most powerful tests you can do within yourself. True fasting brings humility and alignment with the earth we live in and of all the things we can do to enhance our power and focus it is one of the most effective.

Fasting is not easy, and of course, there are degrees of fasting. The physical pain we experience is due to the detoxification of our bodies. All the accumulated poison and rubbish starts to come into our blood and to begin with we feel dreadful. It's a very good lesson, since so many of us use food as an emotional crutch to give pleasure, drowsiness, satisfaction, and/or escape. Fasting instead teaches you to look inside yourself and maybe face other painful issues in your life. Great spiritual victories are won or lost on our willpower and you will experience weakness at times, but it's an amazing feeling in the end to overcome temptation and it leaves us with the feeling of being stronger and more in control. So, whether it means giving up your favourite daily chocolate bar, or not eating every day until lunch time, or a full-on 30-day juice fast, if you can break those emotional ties to the food you love, you will feel better for it.

Get a dose of sea air

Living on the coast improves your health. It's a fact! I always thought my love of the sea was because I grew up living next to the ocean. Surely it's about the mental connection with childhood memories and carefree days? The mere sight of the water calms me and makes me feel happy, and the smell in the air just makes me feel at home.

In fact this is a real thing. Sea air decreases stress and makes you feel great because of the minerals in the air and the negatively charged ions. Sea air contains a significant amount of negatively charged ions which make you feel good. Did you ever notice how you feel better, or even invigorated, after a lightning storm? The reason for this is the release of negative ions. Negative ions are molecules in nature, found in great numbers in places such as the forest or waterfalls. The ocean/sea spray, which is loaded with negative ions, helps strengthen immunological defence mechanisms, and the iodine in the ocean mist helps regulate the thyroid gland, increasing our ability to absorb oxygen and balancing serotonin levels, which are connected to our mood and stress levels, helping us feel happier and healthier.

We are constantly exposed to many positive ions (free radicals) from computers, electricity, television, etc., so this is why it is especially good to increase our exposure to negative ions as much as we possibly can. If you are very brave it's also a fact that individuals who immerse themselves in the cold waters of the ocean at least three times a week increase their white blood cell count, the immune cells that help to fight infection.

Floss before bed

Using dental floss helps to prevent gum disease by removing pieces of food and plaque from between the teeth. If it's left to build up you might notice sore or bleeding gums, and studies have shown links between a build-up of dental plaque and heart disease, Alzheimer's, diabetes, strokes, and lung disease. It's a simple thing that you just need to get in the habit of doing. It takes 30 seconds of your time each day and the health benefits are enormous.

Clean your teeth with charcoal

Years ago, a friend of mine mentioned that his grandmother was 92 and had never had a filling, visited the dentist, or seen a hygienist. When I asked what her secret was, he said that she brushed her teeth with charcoal! I remember being horrified at the time

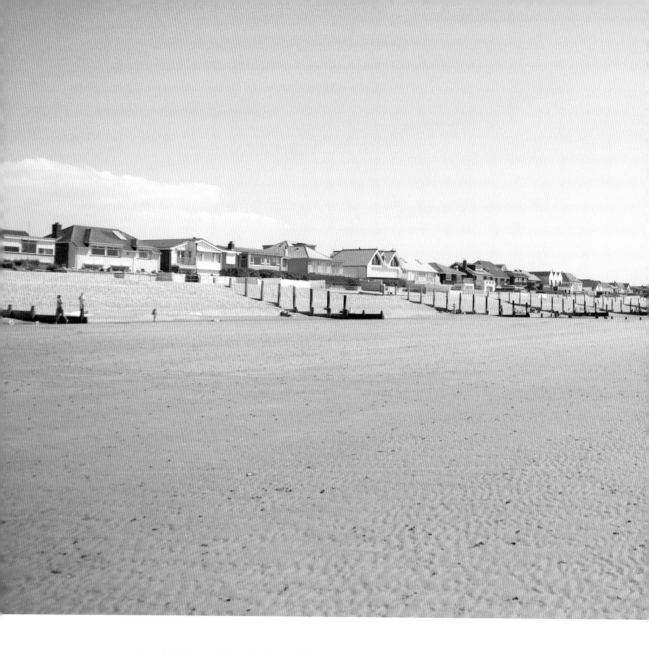

as I couldn't even imagine how disgusting that could be. After I looked into it a little more the idea seemed so positive I wanted to try it out. That was nine years ago and not a day goes by when I don't use charcoal on my teeth. The best thing is that it has removed all the stains, leaves my teeth looking white and gleaming, and I have never had to go to the hygienist again! My gums are healthier than they have ever been – it's honestly a miracle! It can be a little messy, but just brush with care and make sure you don't splash it all over the place if you have a lovely white carpet! The trick is to have two toothbrushes. Use one to dip in your charcoal pot and get the black stuff onto your teeth. Brush as normal. Then secondly get your toothpaste on the clean brush and

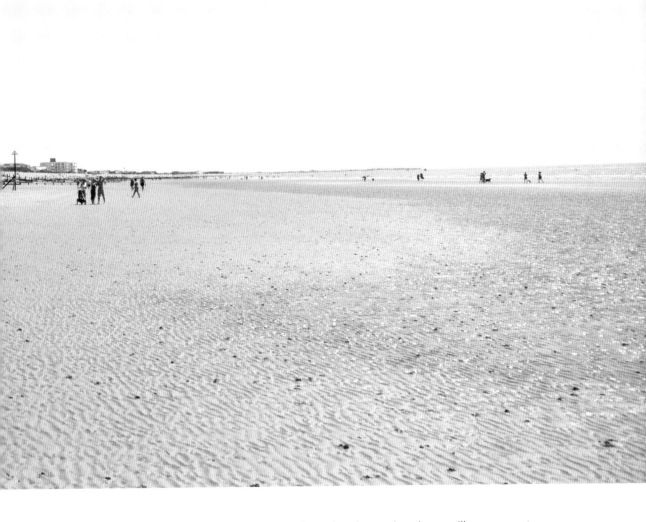

brush as normal. This will remove any black from the charcoal and you will never want to be without it again as your teeth and gums feel wonderful.

Use aromatherapy oils

I go through phases of using aromatherapy oils depending on my mood, and my needs, but I love the natural fragrances that they give off and always find it useful to be reminded of their wonderful benefits. When I go away on holiday I love to take with me the essential oils that I think will be most useful to me and my family, not to mention sprinkling the oils all over the room when I arrive in the apartment or hotel. It just freshens a place up and puts me in the mood for relaxation and fun! Aromatherapy oils should be used with a carrier oil when being applied to the skin, otherwise severe irritation or reaction can occur (and they should not be used during pregnancy). Examples of carrier oils are sweet almond oil, avocado oil, evening primrose oil, hemp seed oil, olive oil, and rose hip oil. Have you noticed a similarity between the carrier oils? They are all good enough to eat, and that's exactly the kind of goodness you want on your skin. I remember someone telling me once, if you would not put it in your mouth, then don't put it on the skin!

Essential/aromatherapy oils are usually distilled from leaves, bark, and roots. Here are my top six:

Frankincense – my favourite of all oils! This is an amazing anti-stress oil used for nervousness, calming the brain, exhaustion, muscle pain, and insomnia. If you or your children are desperate to go to sleep simply rub a pea-sized amount on the soles of your feet.

Grapefruit – great for sickness, constipation, indigestion, nausea, and jet lag.

Lavender – I love the smell of lavender and use it all the time. It's soothing, calming, and wonderful for insomnia. It can be used to treat insect bites, blisters, dry skin, hay fever, headaches, heatstroke, rashes, and sunburn.

Lemon – this is great for the circulation if you have a long haul flight. It's a fabulous disinfectant, and works really well for fatigue, heat exhaustion, jet lag, and feelings of low mood.

Peppermint – fantastic for colds and fevers, heat exposure, heatstroke, sunburn, toothache, nausea, and motion sickness.

Tea tree – this you should always have in your first aid kit, as it's so useful and natural. Amazing for insect bites, blisters, disinfectants, infections, rashes, toothache, wounds, and mouth ulcers. You can use tea tree oil in small amounts directly on the affected area.

With all the oils just place a couple of drops of your desired oil into a palmful of carrier oil and rub into the skin, or burn a few drops in water in a special oil burner to be surrounded by those aromas all day long! So simple, yet so effective and completely natural.

Forgiveness

All of us, without exception, have been emotionally upset by someone, at some point in our lives. Whether it be a partner, mother, brother, father, sister, friend, we all have a story to tell. This is a harsh life lesson to learn, but it is how we deal with it that matters to our bodies in the long term. In order to forgive you must let go of your anger and negative thoughts and forgive the person deep within yourself, as well as outwardly. One of the benefits of forgiveness is lowering the amount of cortisol, therefore lowering the stress levels within our bodies that are so damaging to each and every cell. Forgiveness is also great for the heart – literally lowering both heart rate and blood pressure. Having a forgiving heart may lessen both emotional and physical pain. If you let go of the emotional trauma, chronic pain can actually disappear. It is also said that letting go of anger and applying true forgiveness is linked to significantly reducing your blood pressure.

Laughter

Have you noticed how much children laugh and how natural and, sometimes, how out of control it can be? It's because they have no inhibitions and have the ability to live in the moment and let go! It is a proven fact that laughter creates positive energy amongst groups of people and helps to reduce blood pressure, stimulates the cardiovascular system, reduces muscle tension, and aids the respiratory system by increasing oxygen intake. Laughter increases endorphins, which make us feel happier and since they are the body's natural painkillers, can help decrease moderate to severe pain. Laughter can stimulate the thymus gland, which helps the defence and immune system, protecting us from disease.

Whatever your situation, it seems there is a chemical benefit to the body in finding something to laugh about. Five minutes of laughter each day can cause a whopping 53% increase in your immunity, and even a few minutes of laughter have been found to have the same result as an hour in a relaxation class. Watch a funny movie, go to a comedy show, take your funniest friend out for lunch! Whatever it takes, find a way to laugh every day because it's infectious, contagious, compelling, and the most desirable characteristic mentioned when people are asked what they love most in a partner!

Use natural products for your cleaning

Sparkling kitchens look great, but household cleaning products can cause health problems including rashes, wheezing, asthma, headaches, drowsiness, and general feelings of being unwell. Certain chemical components in cleaning products can be very toxic for the body if breathed in or absorbed through the skin. Using natural products is just as effective and much better for your health. Bicarbonate of soda is fantastic as an abrasive cleaner and also makes a great natural air freshener. Mix some with water and a few drops of essential oil, put in a plant sprayer, and squirt it round the room! Vinegar can also be used to clean windows and surfaces – and lemon juice can remove stains from work tops and leave them looking clean and bright.

Emotional support therapies

Indulge, embark, and involve yourself with whatever therapies work for you. I personally love EFT (emotional freedom technique) because it whips through years of talking and cuts straight to the chase when it comes to emotional issues. It's a series of tapping techniques that you can do on yourself or with the help of a practitioner and is the quickest route to ridding your body of past traumas, events, and stuck emotions. Make sure you find yourself a good therapist with a trusted track record and that they come highly recommended. This is your emotional health we are talking about so do your research. The same goes for counsellors, psychotherapists, and hypnotherapists. In my experience with clients, looking after your emotional health is just as important as looking after your physical body, but the practitioner taking care of you has to be

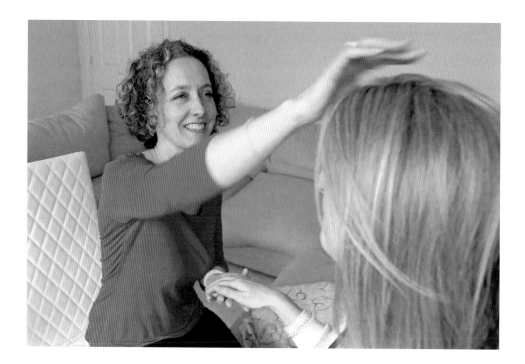

good! Such therapies can give you the strength to grow and learn from each and every experience.

Body work

Osteopathy and acupuncture. Again, in my experience it all comes down to the practitioner. I have met osteopaths with such a natural gift for healing that they give extraordinary treatments. Seeing an osteopath is not just about your back, or your latest neck injury. They are far more than that. They can get you grounded again, help release anxiety and depression, and create straight thinking when your brain feels muddled. I had an ex-serviceman as a client a few years ago, and he had seen some horrific things. He was suffering from PTSD and it had affected his digestion to the point he could hardly eat due to the stress. He had been going from one consultant to another seeking help, and they were running out of answers. I popped him on the health testing machine in my clinic one day, and it was quite clear his diaphragm was restricting his digestion and liver through stress and trauma. Five trips to the osteopath and his digestion was back to normal. He implemented a good clean-living diet and is right as rain to this very day.

When we treat the body holistically, and don't try and separate each organ, we can get far better results, and sometimes the answers are not quite where you have been looking. Acupuncture, reiki, and reflexology are also all great examples of body work treatments you can use to help support and realign your body. Spend time looking after yourself. It is so important.

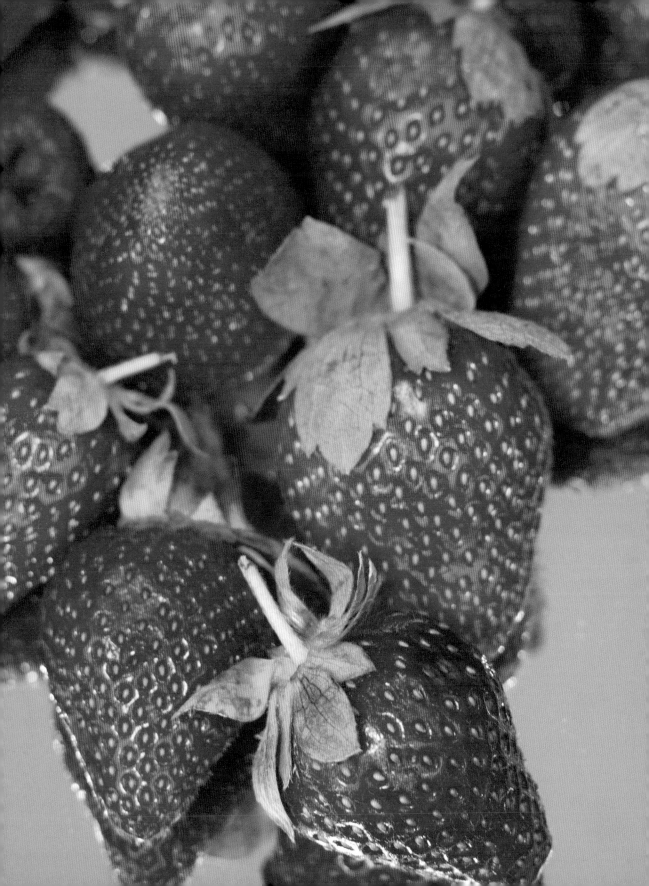

CHAPTER 14

DEVELOP A STRONG LIFE — THE POWER OF YOU

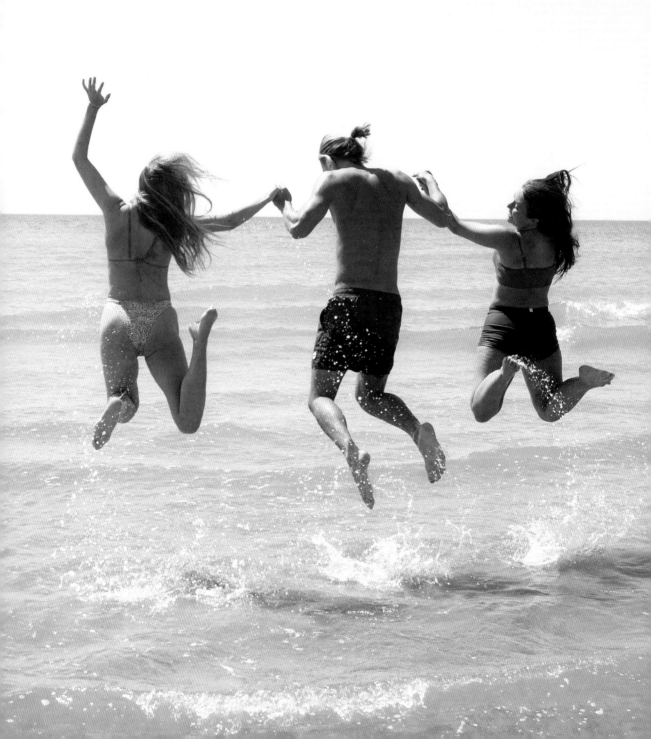

Develop a strong mind and you will live a strong life. A strong mind is built by feeding it with positive thoughts and learning new things every day. When I say this I don't mean every now and then, or perhaps just for a little while, I mean expanding and using the power of your thoughts every single day. Your mind and your soul are like muscles. The more you engage in such practice and awareness, the stronger your understanding will be. If your world is in alignment, things will happen for you naturally. You don't have to fight or force or be desperate for things to change. You actually have to do the opposite. The art in gaining the life you want so much, and creating happiness, abundance, tranquillity, and clarity is to let go. Trust the universe and trust your own process.

Embrace good clean food and healthy living and understand that, as I said before, it isn't about living forever, it's about opening up the possibility of all sorts of incredible opportunities while you are here on this planet and making the best of every single day. I believe if you sit on the sofa all day, drinking, smoking, and eating junk food it clouds your mind, fogs your brain, and numbs your soul. A strong mind is built with daily gratitude and when you are grateful for everything you do there is no room for negativity, and no room for doubt and anxiety. Even if you are in the worst position possible and right at this very moment you feel as if your life couldn't get any lower, then reset your mind. Grab the opportunity with both hands to see how this truly works; after all what do you have to lose?

A strong mind is also built with goals. Goals that give you a reason to get out of bed and seize the day – 'carpe diem' as the roman poet Horace said many times. This basically means enjoying the present and living for the moment. To make the most of today by achieving fulfilment in a philosophical or spiritual sense, attacking the day's efforts with vigour and purpose.

> **You must *stop waiting and start living and make the time for the things you want to do. Say 'yes' to whatever is important and 'no' to what is irrelevant.***

Say 'yes' to what feels right in your heart and 'no' to people that waste your time. Bring your best to the table each and every day and whatever you do, be there fully. Show what you really feel and do not let fear rule you. Be courageous!

Another rule for building a strong mind is accepting that *you* are the only person responsible for your life. Yes pretty ol' you! Not the hunk you hitched up with last week, or your wife or husband you've been with for 30 years, not your children, not your lover, not your best friends. You and only you can make your dreams come true. Your results, your successes, and your failures. And who gives a rat's arse about your failures? I've had loads. Failed marriages, business ideas that didn't work, and no one really remembers them but me. Why? Because everyone is getting on with their world, their bubble of life. And if they do care, and bring you down in any way, send them love – lots of love. There is such power in admitting your mistakes and owning them. Most importantly, continue to learn from your mistakes and expand your mind by developing your skills. Growth is the key to life. If you are growing and challenging yourself every day, you will automatically feel better about yourself. If you are not, you may suffer from loss of confidence. The mind likes to be challenged, it gets stronger when you embrace new things, when you push it to its limits. The more you do this, the better the things you attract. Surrounding yourself with the right people will elevate you and raise your vibration. Do not let the negative opinions of others redirect the course of your life. It follows its own path no matter what. You must visualize what it is you want and be prepared to work to make that picture come true. Do not let fear get in the way and create doubt. If you are determined to learn, no one can stop you.

Be careful of your words, too. Words matter, the words you think, the words you say out loud, and the words that you listen to from others. However, when your words are mixed with your belief, this is when you start noticing shifts in your life and this is what truly creates your reality. What you speak during your life is what your life will become. If you are always talking about how you are stuck, and how you cannot find a way out of the situation that you are in, how you never get any luck, and how you will never be wealthy, you are right, because that is what you will create. If that is what you say, then that is what you believe. Instead of saying 'I don't know how to do it', how about saying 'I am committed to learning how to do it'? Instead of procrastinating and always finding excuses why nothing ever gets done, how about finding something that matters to you more than anything and then deciding and taking action to get the job done?

Instead of saying that you are a failure, say 'I failed, and I have learnt my lessons'. When you become a huge success, it is the failures that make the most interesting of stories. Take Vera Wang, the famous fashion designer, as an example. She wasn't always known for her designer wedding gowns. She was a figure skater that failed to make the US Olympic team. She then moved to work for Vogue but was turned down for the editor-in-chief position before leaving to become the incredible designer she is today. Another fine example is Jeff Bezos, who created Amazon. Before Amazon became a household name, Bezos, had several failed ideas, one being an online auction site, which evolved into ZShops, a brand that ultimately crashed and failed. But with determination and belief, he repurposed the idea into what would eventually become the Amazon Marketplace. Peter Thiel lost 90% of his $7 billion assets invested in the stock market, currencies, and oil. He then started PayPal and invested in names like Facebook to gain greater success than ever before. The list goes on and on. You may be reading this thinking that this is not the kind of success you want at all. My point is always that no matter what you want in life, however big or small, even if it is simply peace and contentment, the same principles apply.

Have you ever heard anyone saying 'My best days are behind me'? What about saying 'My best days are yet to come'? Others are not born lucky or with special gifts, you just need to believe deep in your heart that you are capable of anything. The only limitations that you have are those that you apply to yourself. Your restrictions belong to you, and no one else can do anything about that. Connect with great people, surround yourself with greatness, and become a great person in your own right.

Daily affirmations are so powerful. When you first start to say them, you may feel slightly uncomfortable. But keep repeating them day after day and your mind will start to believe in what you are saying. Start with these and see what happens.

I am a great person	I have no limits
I am a kind person	I have the health and the body of my choice
I am strong	I can have the wealth of my choice
I am capable of anything	I do deserve abundance
I am growing more and more	I am worthy
I am committed	I can make a huge difference in others' lives.
I am determined	

Remember: your beliefs become your thoughts, your thoughts become your words, and your words become your actions. Then your actions become your habits and your habits become your values and your values become your destiny. When you start blending your beliefs and your words together, they become so powerful you can move mountains. You are the creator of your destiny and it starts with the words you speak to yourself and in your life. Bring positive things into your daily practice. Speak love and happiness and abundance and bring them into your life if they're not there already. Speak good of others and avoid negative gossip. Speak your dreams into existence and they will become a reality. Live as if your desires, thoughts, and feelings are real, and they soon will be.

Muhammad Ali said he would be the greatest, and he became the greatest. He had no doubt in his mind, and that is the level of certainty that you should speak about your thoughts, dreams, and desires.

I am healthy, I am wealthy, I am wise.

Opportunities pop up everywhere. Money flows with ease, joy is everywhere, and watch what you are attracting when you vibrate at this level. Feel blessed, surround yourself with blessings. Know that you have more than enough and are full of endless energy. Say to yourself that you are strong and fit and that you are such a positive influence on those around you. Say you have amazing friends, say it all out loud! Say that you are abundant in all areas of your life and that you are constantly growing your income if that's what you want. Say to yourself: I am getting healthier, stronger, and fitter every day and that your relationships are becoming more meaningful and always growing. Say out loud that there is more love and joy every day in your life. Sticks and stones may break your bones, but your words can shatter your dreams.

Your beliefs, thoughts, and dreams will determine your destiny. Whatever you believe is your limit, is your limit. The person you will be in the future is based on everything you do today. The workouts you do, or don't do. The foods you eat today, or don't eat. The books you read, the people you surround yourself with, and the thoughts that feed your mind. Your future self wants you to show some discipline, work hard to achieve your goals. Whatever you want out of life, put the effort in now. If you want success, put the work in, if you want health and fitness, put in the work. If you want peace and happiness, be clear on what you want.

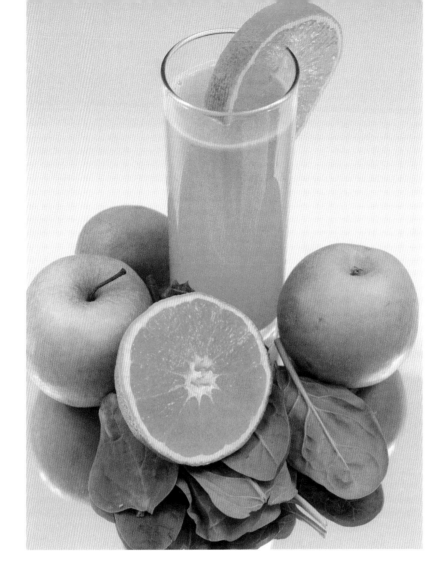

At night-time when you sleep, you are essentially fasting. It gives your body the rest it needs in order to renew and repair your gorgeous cells, but you can use this time for something else too. Recently a client said to me she felt regretful and as if she had wasted the last 10 years of her life being ill, separating from her partner, and not enjoying her job, etc. We can be full of regret, but the most important thing to remember is that every day, every hour, every minute can be a fresh start, so why not use waking up as the perfect opportunity to press your restart button?

Before your feet hit the floor, as soon as thoughts enter your head, make them positive. Stop worrying about things that have been bothering you and allow your energy alignment to take place. Release any feelings of resistance. Go to sleep with gratitude and positivity, and that's how you will wake up. Lay in your bed and appreciate everything and anything that doesn't take you into any negative energy. Think about things that can bring you back into alignment. Bask yourself to sleep with delightful thoughts and then when you wake try to get your immediate thoughts back into the zone that you were in the night before, by reclaiming those happy thoughts. Go right into a list of positive aspects before you start your day. Then your day will be amazing. It takes time, patience, practice, and dedication to do this, but it's so worth it. The results will change your life.

Take whatever you want from this information, run with it, live by it, but I will always stand by my advice to you and say this.

Balance is key in everything you do. You can party all night long if you want to, laugh and be happy, but the next day practise yoga and drink green juice in abundance. Have a chunk of chocolate when you want to, and a bowl of green leaves to keep your body strong when you need to. Put your suit and smart shoes on one day and your trainers the next. Walk barefoot on the grass and then put your stilettos on tomorrow. Love your body whatever your size, shape, or gender. Live high, take risks, be brave, be bold, be spontaneous. Grab opportunities by the horns when they come along. Find your silent peace and be comfortable with who you are. If you are not, then find ways of getting there. Be kind to others always and make time to be kind to yourself. Make your own rules, and follow your own path. This is your life and you deserve only the very best … for you.

THANK YOUS

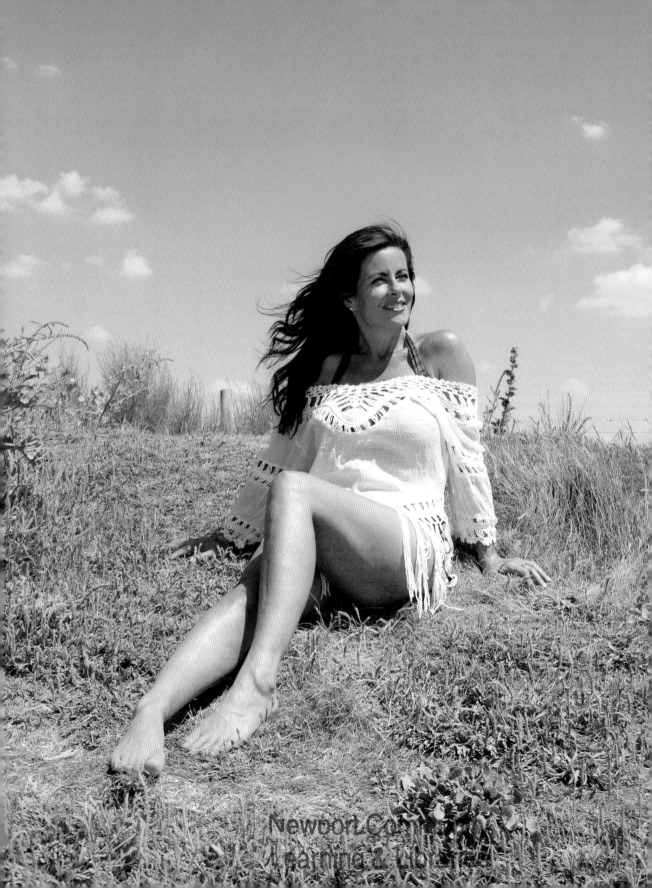

My Bambinos – I cannot really remember life before them! They are my entire world. Emotionally mature and loving way beyond their years, showing me unconditional love and support with whatever crazy idea I embark on next! They teach me lessons every day with their love, laughter, positivity, and happiness. The friendship and protection that they share as brother and sister are all I could ever have wished for, and the strength and bond we have is unbreakable. Thank you for always believing in me, as I do – and always will – in you. I hope I have taught you to think outside the box and follow your heart and your dreams always. You both are the best thing that could ever have happened to me and I am immensely proud and continuously amazed by you. I know things will change as you grow and go on your own adventures over the next few years, but I am beyond excited for you for your next chapters.

My family – I feel so lucky to have to endless support, love, and unwavering dedication from my incredible parents, sister, and extended family which means more than words can ever express. It's a priceless feeling to know you belong and are truly accepted for who you are. Thank you for always being excited and interested in all my ventures and showing me the true meaning of loyalty, strength, and support.

My best friends – you know who you are and without you in my life every day I do not know how I would survive. You make me laugh hysterically until I can't breathe and force me to exercise on a daily basis. We are each other's therapy, and I hope I am as much of a support to you all as you are to me. You show love no matter what and have shown loyalty beyond my wildest dreams. Words cannot express how grateful I am to have you all in my life. I feel blessed every day.

Thank you to the wonderful Bailey Sadler (bnsvisuals.com) who is both talented and creative in his approach to his video and photographic work! He is a blessing in our lives and we are so lucky to have found him! Brilliant and professional.

Thanks to my wonderful and talented friend Catherine Dawtrey (catdphotography.co.uk) for taking some of the photos contained in this book. You're a legend and have more photos dating back to our teenage years than anyone I know!

There are so many other people I would like to thank. People I have learnt from, people who have shown love and kindness over the years, and those who have helped in teaching me new things. The human spirit never fails to surprise and delight me and I am excited for the years ahead. New ventures, new chapters …

About the Author

Denise Kelly has had a colourful career so far in the field of well-being. Her love and passion for health and fitness began when she faced her own health challenges after the birth of her first child, and her nutrition discoveries were to shape the path for her future passion and work. Life has dealt her some real curve balls, but she believes she has come out stronger and more robust because of those challenges.

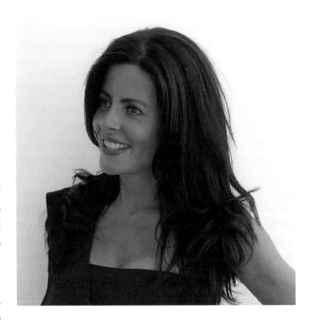

She runs busy clinics in the UK where she sees clients on a one to one basis helping them overcome and improve their health with personalized nutrition planning and well-being advice. She has spoken all over the world at health conferences and corporate events on the subject of energy and wellness and writes for many corporate organizations as well as being a columnist for individual papers.

Denise is an entrepreneur, turning many ideas and passions into businesses, but also gives up her time to help teach how to become healthier within charity organizations. She has a busy family life, and truly believes 'life is for thriving and not just surviving'. Her goal is to reach as many people as possible in the world to help them discover how to be the best version of themselves. She believes that our whole functioning depends on the food we eat, the air we breathe, the movement in our bodies, the people we surround ourselves with and our attitude to life. She truly believes that focusing on improving health, enhances your life in all areas, be it career, family, love, sport, fitness etc., and that anything is possible!

If you want any of the products discussed in this book or need nutritional information please visit **www.denisekelly.co.uk**

INDEX